THOMSON DELMAR LEARNING'S
NURSING REVIEW SERIES

Gerontologic Nursing

THOMSON DELMAR LEARNING'S NURSING REVIEW SERIES

LIBRARY OF
Methodist
College of Nursing

Gerontologic Nursing

Content taken from:
Delmar's Complete Review for NCLEX-RN®

By:
Donna F. Gauwitz, RN, MS
Nursing Consultant
Former Senior Teaching Specialist
School of Nursing
University of Minnesota Twin Cities
Minneapolis, Minnesota
Former Nursing Education Specialist
Mayo Clinic
Rochester, Minnesota

THOMSON
*
DELMAR LEARNING   Australia   Canada   Mexico   Singapore   Spain   United Kingdom   United States

THOMSON

DELMAR LEARNING

Nursing Review Series: Gerontologic Nursing

by Donna F. Gauwitz

Vice President, Health Care Business Unit:
William Brottmiller

Director of Learning Solutions:
Matthew Kane

Acquisitions Editor:
Tamara Caruso

Product Manager:
Patricia Gaworecki

Editorial Assistant:
Jenn Waters

Marketing Director:
Jennifer McAvey

Marketing Channel Manager:
Michele McTighe

Marketing Coordinator:
Danielle Pacella

Technology Director:
Laurie Davis

Technology Project Manager:
Mary Colleen Liburdi
Patricia Allen

Production Director:
Carolyn Miller

Production Manager:
Barbara Bullock

Art Director:
Robert Plante
Jack Pendleton

Content Project Manager:
Dave Buddle
Stacey Lamodi
Jessica McNavich

Production Coordinator:
Mary Ellen Cox

Library of Congress Cataloging-
in-Publication Data
ISBN 1-4018-1181-7

Notice to the Reader

Contents

Contributors

Mary Mescher Benbenek, RN, MS, CPNP, CFNP
Teaching Specialist
School of Nursing
University of Minnesota
Twin Cities, Minnesota

Margaret Brogan, RN, BSN
Registered Nurse/Expert
Children's Memorial Hospital
Chicago, Illinois

Mary Lynn Burnett, RN, PhD
Assistant Professor of Nursing
Wichita State University
Wichita, Kansas

Corine K. Carlson, RN, MS
Assistant Professor
Department of Nursing
Luther College
Decorah, Iowa

Gretchen Reising Cornell, RN, PhD, CNE
Professor of Nursing
Utah Valley State College
Orem, Utah

Vera V. Cull, RN, DSN
Former Assistant Professor of Nursing
University of Alabama
Birmingham, Alabama

Laura DeHelian, RN, PhD, APRN, BC
Former Assistant Professor of Nursing
Cleveland State University
Cleveland, Ohio

Della J. Derscheid, RN, MS, CNS
Assistant Professor
Department of Nursing
Mayo Clinic
Mayo Clinic College of Nursing
Rochester, Minnesota

Ann Garey, MSN, APRN, BC, FNP
Carle Foundation Hospital
Urbana, Illinois

Beth Good, RN, MSN, BSN
Teaching Specialist
University of Minnesota
Minneapolis, Minnesota

Samantha Grover, RN, BSN, CNS
Psychiatric Mental Health Clinical Specialist
MeritCare Health System
Moorhead, Minnesota

Jeanne M. Harkness, RN, BA, MSN, BSN, AOCN
Clinical Practice Specialist
Jane Brattain Breast Center
Park Nicollet Clinic
St. Louis Park, Minnesota

Linda Irle, RN, MSN, APN, CNP
Coordinator, Maternal-Child Nursing
University of Illinois
Urbana, Illinois
Family Nurse Practitioner, Acute Care,
Carle Clinic,
Champaign, Illinois

Amy Jacobson, RN, BA
Staff Nurse
United Hospital
St. Paul, Minnesota

Nadine James, RN, PhD
Assistant Professor of Nursing
University of Southern Mississippi
Hattiesburg, Mississippi

Lisa Jensen, CS, MS, APRN
Salt Lake City VA Healthcare System
Salt Lake City, Utah

Ellen Joswiak, RN, MA
Assistant Professor of Nursing
Staff Nurse
Mayo Medical Center
Rochester, Minnesota

Betsy Ann Skrha Kennedy, RN, MS,
CS, LCCE
Nursing Instructor
Rochester Community and Technical
    College
Rochester, Minnesota

Robin M. Lally, PhD, RN, BA, AOCN, CNS
Teaching Specialist; Office 6-155
School of Nursing
University of Minnesota
Twin Cities, Minnesota

Penny Leake, RN, PhD
Luther College
Decorah, Iowa

Barbara Mandleco, RN, PhD
Associate Professor & Undergraduate
    Program Coordinator
College of Nursing
Brigham Young University
Provo, Utah

Gerry Matsumura, RN, PhD, MSN, BSN
Former Associate Professor of Nursing
Brigham Young University
Provo, Utah

Alberta McCaleb, RN, DSN
Associate Professor
Chair, Undergraduate Studies
University of Alabama School of Nursing
University of Alabama at Birmingham
Birmingham, Alabama

JoAnn Mulready-Shick, RN, MS
Dean, Nursing and Allied Health
Roxbury Community College
Boston, Massachusetts

Patricia Murdoch, RN, MS
Nurse Practitioner
University of Illinois, Chicago
Urbana, Illinois

Jayme S. Nelson, RN, MS, ARNP-C
Adult Nurse Practitioner
Assistant Professor of Nursing
Luther College
Decorah, Iowa

Janice Nuuhiwa, MSN, CPON, APN/
CNS
Staff Development Specialist
Hematology/Oncology/Stem Cell
    Transplant Division
Children's Memorial Hospital
Chicago, Illinois

Kristen L. Osborn, MSN, CRNP
Pediatric Nurse Specialist
UAB School of Nursing
UAB Pediatric Hematology/Oncology
Birmingham, Alabama

Karen D. Peterson, RN, MSN, BSN, PNP
Pediatric Nurse Practitioner
Division of Endocrinology
Children's Memorial Hospital
Chicago, Illinois

Kristin Sandau, RN, PhD
Bethel University's Department of
    Nursing
United's John Nasseff Heart Hospital
Minneapolis, Minnesota

Elizabeth Sawyer, RN, BSN, CCRN
Registered Nurse
United Hospital
St. Paul, Minnesota

Lisa A. Seldomridge, RN, PhD
Associate Professor of Nursing
Salisbury University
Salisbury, Maryland

Janice L. Vincent, RN, DSN
University of Alabama School of Nursing
University of Alabama at Birmingham
Birmingham, Alabama

Margaret Vogel, RN, MSN, BSN
Nursing Instructor
Rochester Community & Technical
   College
Rochester, Minnesota

Mary Shannon Ward, RN, MSN
Children's Memorial Hospital
Chicago, Illinois

Preface

Congratulations on discovering the best new review series for the NCLEX-RN®! Thomson Delmar Learning's Nursing Review Series is designed to maximize your study in the core subject areas covered on the NCLEX-RN® examination. The series consists of 8 books:

Pharmacology

Medical-Surgical Nursing

Pediatric Nursing

Maternity and Women's Health Nursing

Gerontologic Nursing

Psychiatric Nursing

Legal and Ethical Nursing

Community Health Nursing

Each text has been developed expressly to meet your needs as you study and prepare for the all-important licensure examination. Taking this exam is a stressful event and constitutes a major career milestone. Passing the NCLEX is the key to your future ability to practice as a registered nurse.

Each text in the series is designed around the most current test plan for the NCLEX-RN® and provides a focused and complete content review in each subject area. Additionally, there are up to 400 review questions in each text: questions at the end of most every chapter and three 100 question review tests that support the chapter content. Each set of review questions is followed by answers and rationales for both the right and wrong answers. There is also a free PDA download of review questions available with the purchase of any of these review texts! It is this combination of content review and self assessment that provides a powerful learning experience for you as you prepare for you examination.

ORGANIZATION

Thomson Delmar Learning's unique Pharmacology review book provides you with an intensive review in this all important subject area. Drugs are grouped by classification and similarities to aid you in consolidating this pertinent but sometimes overwhelming information. Included in this text are:

- A section on herbal medicines, now being tested on the exam.
- Case studies that apply relevant drug content
- Prototypes for most drug classifications
- Mechanism of drug action
- Uses and adverse effects
- Nursing implications and discharge teaching
- Related drugs and their variance from the prototype

The review texts for Medical-Surgical Nursing, Pediatric Nursing, Maternity Nursing, Gerontological Nursing and Psychiatric Nursing follow a systematic approach that includes:

- The nursing process integrated with a body systems approach
- Introductory review of normal anatomy and physiology as well as basic theories and principles
- Review of pertinent disorders for each system including: general characteristics, pathophysiology/psychopathology
- Medical management
- Assessment data
- Nursing interventions and client education

Community Health Nursing and Legal and Ethical Nursing are unique review texts in the marketplace. They include aspects of community health nursing and legal/ethical subject matter that is covered on the NCLEX-RN® exam. Community Health topics covered are: case management, long-term care, home health care and hospice. Legal and ethical topics include: cultural diversity, leadership and management, ethical issues and legal issues for older adults.

FEATURES

All questions in each text in the series are compliant with the most current test plan from the National Council of State Boards of Nursing (NCSBN). All questions are followed by answers and rationales for both right and wrong choices. Included are many of the alternative format questions first introduced to the exam in 2003. An icon identifies these alternate types ⊙. The questions in each of these texts are written primarily at the application or analysis cognitive levels allowing you to further enhance critical thinking skills which are heavily weighted on the NCLEX.

In addition, with the purchase of any of these texts, a free PDA download is available to you. It provides you with up to an additional 225 questions with which you can practice your test taking skills.

Thomson Delmar Learning is committed to help you reach your fullest professional potential. Good luck on the NCLEX-RN® examination!

> To access your free PDA download for Thomson Delmar Learning's Nursing Review Series visit the online companion resource at **www.delmarhealthcare.com** Click on Online Companions then select the Nursing discipline.

Reviewers

Dr. Geri Beers, RN, EdD
Associate Professor of Nursing
Samford University
Birmingham, Alabama

Nancy D. Bingaman, RN, MS
Nursing Instructor
Maurine Church Coburn School of
    Nursing
Monterey Peninsula College
Monterey, California

Carol Boswell, EdD, RN
Associate Professor
College of Nursing
Texas Tech University Health Sciences
    Center
Odessa, Texas

Judy A. Bourrand, RN, MSN
Assistant Professor
Ida V. Moffett School of Nursing
Samford University
Birmingham, Alabama

Clara Willard Boyle, RN, BS, MS, EdD
Associate Professor
Salem State College
Salem, Massachusetts

Rebecca Gesler, MSN, RN
Assistant Professor
Spalding University
Louisville, Kentucky

Susan Hinck, PhD, RN, CS
Associate Professor
Department of Nursing
Missouri State University
Springfield, Missouri

Mary M. Hoke, PhD, APRN-BC
Academic Department Head
New Mexico State University
Las Cruces, New Mexico

Loretta J. Heuer, PhD, RN, FAAN
Associate Professor
College of Nursing
University of North Dakota
Grand Forks, North Dakota

Ann Putnam Johnson, EdD, RN
Professor of Nursing
Associate Dean, College of Applied
    Sciences
Western Carolina University
Cullowhee, North Carolina

Brenda P. Johnson, PhD, RN
Associate Professor, Dept. of Nursing
Southeast Missouri State
    University
Cape Girardeau, Missouri

Pat. S. Kupina, RN, MSN
Professor of Nursing
Joliet Junior College
Joliet, Illinois

Mary Lashley, RN, PhD, APRN, BC
Associate Professor
Department of Nursing
Towson University
Towson, Maryland

Melissa Lickteig, EdD, RN
Assistant Professor
School of Nursing
Georgia Southern University
Statesboro, Georgia

Caron Martin, MSN, RN
Associate Professor
School of Nursing and Health
   Professions
Northern Kentucky University
Highland Heights, Kentucky

Darlene Mathis, MSN, RN, APRN, BC, NP-C, CNE, CRNP
Assistant Professor and Certified Nurse
   Educator
Samford University Ida V. Moffett School
   of Nursing
Family Nurse Practitioner
Birmingham Health Care
Birmingham, Alabama

Carol E. Meadows, MNSc, RNP, APN
Instructor
Eleanor Mann School of Nursing
University of Arkansas
Fayetteville, Arkansas

Margaret A. Miklancie, PhD, RN
Assistant Professor
College of Nursing & Health Science
George Mason University
Fairfax, Virginia

Frances D. Monahan, PhD, RN
Professor of Nursing
SUNY Rockland Community
   College
Consutant, Excelsior College

Deb Poling, MSN, APRN, BC, FNP, ANP
Assistant Professor
Regis University
Denver, Colorado
Case Manager
The Childrens Hospital
Denver, Colorado

Abby Selby, MNSc, RN
Faculty
Mental Health and Illness
Eleanor Mann School of Nursing
College of Education and Health Professions
University of Arkansas
Fayetteville, Arkansas
PRN educator
Mental Health Topics
Northwest Health System
Springdale, Arkansas

Sarah E. Shannon, PhD, RN
Associate Professor
Biobehavioral Nursing and Health Systems
Adjunct Associate Professor
Medical History and Ethics
University of Washington
Seattle, Washington

Susan Sienkiewicz, MA, RN
Professor
Community College of Rhode Island
Warwick, Rhode Island

Maria A. Smith, DSN, RN, CCRN
Professor
School of Nursing
Middle Tennessee State University
Murfreesboro, Tennessee

Ellen Stuart, MSN, RN
Professor
Mental Health Nursing
Grand Rapids Community College
Grand Rapids, Michigan

Karen Gahan Tarnow, RN, PhD
Faculty
School of Nursing
University of Kansas
Kansas City, Kansas

Janice Tazbir, RN, MS, CCRN
Associate Professor of Nursing
School of Nursing
Purdue University Calumet
Hammond, Indiana

Patricia C. Wagner, MSN, RNC
Clinical Assistant Professor
MCN Department, College of Nursing
University of South Alabama
Mobile, Alabama

Health Issues of the Older Adult

■ THEORIES OF AGING

A. Biological Theories
   1. Aging is different among humans.
   2. Aging is different among body systems.
   3. Aging and disease are not synonymous.
   4. Older adults should be encouraged to continue their daily activities.
   5. Genetic Factors.
      a. Genetic program or biological clock predetermines life.
      b. Senescence under genetic control at cellular level
      c. Mutations tend to cause organ decline.
   6. Cross-Linking
      a. Cellular division is altered by chemical reactions.
      b. Cross-linking agents obstruct intracellular transport, leading to failure of body organs.
   7. Free radicals
      a. Free radicals replace molecules with useful biological information with faulty information, causing genetic disorders.
      b. As molecules accumulate, there is a physical decline.
      c. The effects of free radicals are counteracted by natural body oxidants.
   8. Autoimmune Reactions
      a. Thyroid, bone marrow, and immune system are affected by the aging process.
      b. Decrease in thymus and a deterioration in the immune response
      c. Decrease in production of T-cell differentiation
      d. An increase in infections and cancers results in changes.
   9. Wear and tear
      a. Cells wear out over an individual's life.
      b. Repeated injuries, trauma, or stress may increase the process of aging.
B. Psychological Theories
   1. Influenced by biology and sociology
   2. Includes behavioral and developmental aspects of life

3. Adaptive processes such as memory, learning capacity, feelings, intellectual functioning, and motivations guide the older adult to make some biological changes.
4. Past accomplishments are incorporated into life to promote self-esteem.
5. Intellectual functioning remains intact for the majority of adults.
6. Maslow's hierarchy of human needs
7. Erickson's Theory
    a. Ego integrity versus despair
    b. Older adult is concerned with guiding the next generation.
    c. Unsuccessful resolution may result in despair.
C. Sociologic Theories
    1. Focuses on roles and relationship
    2. Societal values may define view of self.
    3. Older adults are individuals.
    4. Responses of older adults should be respected.
    5. Realistic activities should be planned to increase self-confidence.
    6. Older adults should be assisted in their adaptation to their limitations.
    7. Disengagement
        a. Mutual agreement between the older adult and society is withdrawn from society.
        b. Instead of interacting with society, older adults may become self-centered.
    8. Activity
        a. A positive self-concept is necessary to maintain life satisfaction.
        b. The older adult should not withdraw from society.
    9. Continuity
        a. The older adult should be encouraged to continue with the same lifestyle.
        b. Maintains values, beliefs, and commitments that contributes to Personalities

■ NURSING DIAGNOSES

The older adult's physical, psychological, and societal well-being may adversely affect any body system resulting in any possible nursing diagnosis, such as impaired physical mobility, impaired memory, imbalanced nutrition, less than body requirements, self-care deficit, and social isolation.

■ EFFECTS OF AGING ON THE BODY SYSTEMS

A. Respiratory System
    1. Alterations in Anatomy and Physiology
        a. The lungs of an older adult are less flexible and compliant.
        b. Inspiratory and tidal volume decrease with age.
        c. Aging decreases the flexibility of the ribs and weakens chest wall muscles so that inspiration is not as deep.

NURSING ALERT

T he RN should stress the importance of flu and pneumonia immunization to geriatric clients.

DELEGATION TIP

W hen delegating tasks such as assisting a geriatric client with meals, the RN must explain not to rush the client because it may increase shortness of breath and put the client at risk for aspiration.

      d. Atrophy of cilia
      e. Decreased and thickened alveoli
  2. Assessment
      a. Barrel chest
      b. Decreased cough reflex
      c. Increased infection
      d. Difficulty deep breathing
      e. Decreased sensitivity to hypoxia and hypercapnia
      f. Comorbidity may adversely affect gas exchange and airway clearance, resulting in chronic obstructive pulmonary disease (COPD), emphysema with a decrease in tidal volume, asthma, chronic bronchitis, pulmonary fibrosis, tuberculosis, and rarer conditions such as pneumocystis pneumonia.
  3. Diagnostic Tests
      a. Chest x-ray
      b. Oxygen saturation
      c. Biopsy
      d. Sputum culture and sensitivity
      e. CT scan
      f. Sleep evaluation to identify sleep apnea
  4. Nursing Interventions
      a. Auscultate all lung fields anteriorly and posteriorly.
      b. Observe for color and capillary refill.
      c. Utilize pulse oximetry to measure O_2 saturation (expected saturation is 90-100% on room air.
          1) The O_2 saturation may be lower at higher altitudes in the older adult.

NURSING ALERT

The geriatric client may not be able to lie flat for tests or procedures. You should alert others of this consideration when scheduling clients for procedures.

2) Oxygen therapy is necessary only if the client is symptomatic such as having shortness of breath, increased respiratory and heart rates.

d. Assess for shortness of breath and dyspnea on exertion.

e. Ask the client, "What is the hardest thing you do every day?" to assess for fatigue and quality of life.

f. Monitor arterial blood gases, if indicated, evaluating for a decreased PaO_2 and increased $PaCO_2$ (the closer together they become, the more serious the client's condition).

g. Observe sputum for color and presence of blood.

h. Observe how fatigue and shortness of breath affect nutritional intake.

i. Schedule activities to prevent extreme fatigue.

j. Administer oxygen generally by nasal cannula at 2–3 L/min to the client with chronic lung conditions. A higher flow rate will depress the respiratory drive.

k. Sequence activities to promote quality of life, such as a shower in a shower chair at night, so that the oxygen requirements for bathing will not interfere with food digestion as it would earlier in the day.

l. Provide for comfort such as oxygen administration and head of the bed elevated (client may prefer to sleep in a reclining chair or with an electric fan blowing to increase air circulation).

m. Provide small frequent nutrient dense feedings. If the client's CO_2 level is high, then the intake of carbohydrates may be decreased (carbohydrates are metabolized to produce CO_2 and water).

n. Offer fluid intake to 2,000–3,000 ml. a day unless contraindicated.

o. Schedule medications such as non steroidal bronchodilators so that they do not interfere with rest periods because they have a adverse reaction of insomnia. These also increase heart and respiratory rate as well as blood pressure.

p. Monitor the client for infection if taking steroids such as anti-inflammatory medications.

q. Provide for immunizations for diseases that could be fatal for the client with a compromised respiratory system such as influenza and pneumonia.

CLIENT TEACHING CHECKLIST

Geriatric clients and their caregivers should know signs of pulmonary infections:

- Fever, but often baseline temperatures are lower in the geriatric population
- Increased shortness of breath
- Change in level of consciousness or increased confusion
- Increased sputum production or change in color of sputum

     r. Instruct the client about smoking cessation and avoidance of inhaled pollutants, such as wood smoke from a fireplace or aerosol sprays.

     s. Instruct the client's family member how to perform postural drainage and clapping if prescribed.

        1) It is difficult for the older adult to assume the necessary positions.

        2) The family member may also be an older adult who does not have the strength to perform the treatment due to arthritis or chronic conditions

B. Circulation

  1. Alterations in Anatomy and Physiology

    a. Decreased strength of ventricular contraction

    b. Decreased ejection fraction

    c. Arteries become less pliable.

    d. Less sensitive baroreceptors

    e. Thick and rigid heart valves such as aortic and mitral values

    f. Decline in pacemaker cells

  2. Assessment

    a. Varicose veins

    b. Hypertension

    c. Stenosis or insufficiency of heart valves

    d. Orthostatic hypotension

    e. Increased edema in dependent body parts

    f. Heart murmurs

    g. Dysrhythmias

    h. Comorbid conditions may cause serious cardiovascular problems such as diabetes mellitus, hypercholesterolemia, anemia, coronary artery disease, peripheral vascular disorders, congestive heart failure, conduction disorders, and dysrhythmias.

  3. Diagnostic Tests

    a. C reactive protein

    b. Complete blood count

    c. Cholesterol (HDL and LDL) and triglyceride levels
    d. Echocardiogram (external and esophageal)
    e. Electrocardiogram
 4. Nursing Interventions
    a. Monitor blood pressure, heart rate and rhythm, cholesterol and triglyceride levels, oxygen saturation percentages, peripheral circulation, and renal function.
    b. Monitor skin color, temperature, and any discolorations.
    c. Monitor the client for changes in mental status such as confusion, which may be the result of an alteration in oxygenation. (Pneumonia or a myocardial infarction may present with confusion in the older adult.)
    d. Palpate the radial and pedal pulses.
    e. Auscultate pedal, apical, abdominal aorta and carotid pulses by Doppler if appropriate
    f. Assess blood pressure while lying, sitting, and standing.
    g. Instruct the client to stay warm with socks, gloves, and blankets rather than the use of external heat such as heating pads or heat lamps, which may cause burns.
    h. Assess for changes in mental status or cognition. An older adult experiencing a myocardial infarction may become agitated or nauseated because of the decreased perfusion without chest pain.
    i. Instruct the client or family member of any specific assessments needed related to medication administration such as taking a pulse for 1 full minute before administering digitalis preparations and notifying the physician if the pulse is less than 60 or over 100.
    j. Instruct the client's family member how to take, record, and report a blood pressure, and how to inspect the client's feet for alterations in circulation.
C. Elimination
 1. Alterations in Anatomy and Physiology
    a. Slowed gastrointestinal peristalsis
    b. Decreased absorption of nutrients from the gastrointestinal tract
    c. Decreased smooth muscle tone

CLIENT TEACHING CHECKLIST

Teach geriatric clients concerning medications and elimination:

- Medications that increase urination should be scheduled to be taken when client will have access to the bathroom.
- Medications that cause diarrhea will increase fluid needs.
- Medications that cause constipation will increase the need for fluid, fiber, and exercise.

      d. Weakened muscles used in swallowing
      e. Decrease in gastric enzymes
      f. Decreased sphincter tone
2. Assessment
      a. Decreased gastrointestinal motility
      b. Difficulty swallowing
      c. Heartburn
      d. Constipation
      e. Loss of teeth
      f. Decreased saliva
      g. Decreased taste
      h. Malabsorption
      i. Comorbid conditions that affect elimination patterns are those that primarily decrease mobility such as arthritis or a CVA, or decrease fluid intake such as dementia or renal failure.
3. Diagnostic Tests
      a. Urinalysis with culture and sensitivity
      b. Stool specimen for ova, parasites, and fecal fat
      c. Stool specimen for occult blood
      d. Colonoscopy
      e. Barium swallow or barium enema, or both
4. Nursing Interventions
      a. Assess for an increased urinary output if the client is taking diuretics.
      b. Assess for diarrhea if the client is taking antibiotics.
      c. Monitor a male client who has benign prostatic hypertrophy for urinary frequency in small amounts of urine and nocturia.
      d. Monitor a female client for urinary incontinence that may occur as a result of having had many vaginal deliveries or cystocele.
      e. Assess for types of incontinence such as urge, stress, and neurogenic.

NURSING ALERT

I f you determine elimination patterns in the geriatric client, you may be proactive and work with elimination issues before they become problematic for the client.

DELEGATION TIP

Y ou should teach assistive personnel to be sensitive to the geriatric client's elimination needs and promptly answer call lights to avoid use of incontinence pads.

    f.   Assess for constipation or perceived constipation. These may result in self-medications with over-the-counter (OTC) preparations. Laxative abuse can occur when the clients expectations for bowel movement regularity are not met.

    g.   Monitor the client's urine for color, clarity, amount, and any inclusions. An older adult may not have the ability or the vision to be an accurate reporter.

    h.   Evaluate the client's daily fluid intake. The client may intentionally limit fluids in order to decrease trips to the toilet, especially if taking a diuretic.

    i.   Evaluate the client's bowel elimination. Determine the client's definition of what are "normal" bowel movements. Identify OTC medications and methods used for regularity.

    j.   Monitor bowel movements for color, consistency, amount, and frequency.

    k.   Administer stool softeners, prune juice, fiber, and increased fluid intake for constipation.

    l.   Administer laxatives if other methods for regularity fail, using enemas infrequently.

    m.   Provide for regular toileting usually after breakfast.

    n.   Implement a toileting schedule to prevent urinary incontinence. Incontinence may be not only embarrassing for the client but also a cause of social isolation, depression, and falls after hurrying to the toilet or slipping on a wet floor.

    o.   Instruct the client to avoid caffeine and alcohol in the presence of urinary incontinence.

    p.   Instruct the client on the importance of adequate (2,000–3,000 ml per day) intake of oral fluids and a diet rich in fiber.

NURSING ALERT

G eriatric clients may have altered pain perception and may not report intense pain with fractures.

    q. Assess a client with a urinary tract infection for confusion, incontinence, and anorexia rather than a fever, frequency, and urgency.

D. Mobility
1. Alterations in Anatomy and Physiology
   a. Without use muscles decrease in size and strength.
   b. Decreased bone density
   c. Tendons and ligaments lose elasticity.
   d. Narrowed intervertebral disks
2. Assessment
   a. Weak
   b. Reduced range of motion
   c. Unsteady balance, which may be compounded by inner ear problems, electrolyte imbalances, dehydration, anemia, and muscle weakness
   d. Osteoporosis results from inadequate calcium intake, inadequate Vitamin D synthesis or ingestion, lack of weight bearing, medications (such as corticosteroids), or smoking. As the bones weaken, the older adult is at risk for falls, fractures, kyphosis, and compression of vertebrae.
   e. Slowed gait because of chronic and degenerative conditions such as osteoarthritis, bunions, or obesity.
3. Diagnostic Tests.
   a. Creatinine phosphokinase CPK to identify muscle activity
   b. Serum electrolytes
   c. X-rays, bone scans, and CT scans for skeletal anomalies
   d. Assessment of balance and gait
4. Nursing Interventions
   a. Monitor electrolytes, fluid balance, blood counts, and ability to perform activities of daily living (ADLs).
   b. Assess muscle strength, gait, and balance.
   c. Complete a functional assessment profile.
   d. Identify the client's fall risk.
      1) Determine if shoes fit adequately.
      2) The presence of hazards in the home such as pets on the floor, throw rugs, clutter, electrical cords, and oxygen administration tubing

NURSING ALERT

P romoting activities that stimulate the mind, such as reading or crossword puzzles, may help geriatric clients' neurological function.

  e. Assess for consequences of immobility and institute preventive measures.
   1) Adequate hydration and leg exercises to prevent deep vein thrombosis and pulmonary embolism
   2) Range of motion exercises to maintain muscle tone and prevent weakness
   3) Adequate exercise to prevent insomnia
   4) Diversional activities and social stimulation to prevent loneliness and depression
   5) Weight bearing as appropriate and calcium (1200–1500 mg/day) to prevent osteoporosis.
   6) Adequate fluid intake (2000–3000 ml./day) to prevent hemoconcentration, urinary tract infection, constipation, and urinary lithiasis.
   7) Adequate pain control so that the client is able to be mobile
   8) Monitor bowel movements and ensure adequate intake of fiber and fluids to prevent constipation.
   9) Observe skin frequently and prevent breakdown by providing position changes every 2 hours, adequate protein intake, and adequate fluid intake.
E. Neurological Function
 1. Alterations in Anatomy and Physiology
  a. Decreased reflexes
  b. Decreased blood flow to the brain
  c. Deterioration of the myelin sheath
  d. The actual size of the brain in the normal older adult will decrease in size and weight by up to one-third.
 2. Assessment
  a. Sluggish reflexes
  b. Short-term memory problems
  c. Confusion
  d. Decreased ability to learn
 3. Diagnostic Tests
  a. Myelogram
  b. CT scan or other noninvasive scans
  c. Spinal tap
  d. Carotid or cerebral arteriogram

4. Nursing Interventions
    a. Caution the older adult that she may have a slowed response while operating a motor vehicle.
    b. Monitor the client for short-term memory problems.
    c. Assess the client for atherosclerosis, hypertension, or transient ischemic attacks.
    d. Monitor cognition, level of consciousness, pupils, cranial nerves, and peripheral nerve function.
    e. Assess sensation and motor function.
    f. Evaluate the effect of medications on neurological function such as an impairment in self-care deficit.

F. Sensory Function
    1. Alteration in Anatomy and Physiology
        a. Vision changes from nearsightedness (myopia) to farsightedness (presbyopia) in most adults
        b. Decreased blood supply to the ear
        c. Slowed pupil accommodation
        d. Atrophied olfactory fibers
        e. Decreased lacrimal secretions
        f. Larger, discolored, and more rigid lens
    2. Assessment
        a. Decreased taste and smell
        b. Decreased ability to distinguish item in the hands or on the feet
        c. Decreased hearing
        d. Increased sensitivity to glare
        e. Dry eyes
        f. Decreased ability to focus on objects
        g. Decreased ability to distinguish between sounds
        h. Decreased depth perception
        i. Excess wax production
    3. Diagnostic Tests
        a. Tympanography
        b. Evaluation of cranial nerves
        c. Vision evaluation with measurement of intraocular pressure, optic nerve, and retina
        d. Evaluation of visual fields
    4. Nursing Interventions
        a. Question the client related to loud prolonged noises earlier in life, such as rock music or machinery in the workplace.
        b. Assess the pupils and inform the client to avoid night driving because pupil accommodation slows.
        c. Inform the client that food may not taste as good.
        d. Assess the client for comorbid conditions that may pose serious safety risks for the older adult.

NURSING ALERT

Y ou should be alert to assess the hearing impaired client's home environment to ensure that fire alarms and phones can be heard.

NURSING ALERT

D riving is often synonymous with independence in the geriatric client. The issue of driving restrictions should be dealt with great sensitivity to autonomy.

1) Glaucoma—increase in intraocular pressure and decrease in peripheral vision leading to total loss of vision if untreated
2) Macular degeneration—loss of central vision
3) Cataracts—opacity of the lens that is so gradual that the client may be unaware of decreasing vision. Leads to blindness but lens can be replaced surgically and vision restored.
4) Diabetes mellitus—retinopathy which leads to blindness. The loss of vision can be prevented by maintaining blood glucose levels within normal range.

   e. Evaluate ability to hear, and inspect the ear canal for excess wax buildup.
   f. Assess vision, ability to read printed instructions, and inspect the eye and lids.
   g. Evaluate the range of odors that the client can recognize, focusing on the priority, which is the ability to recognize smoke in the environment.
   h. Identify risks posed by sensory limitations.
   i. Instruct the client on information vital to preventing further deterioration of eyesight, such as prescribed eyedrops for glaucoma that constrict the pupils and must be used for the rest of her life, and to maintain blood sugar within the normal limits.
G. Integumentary System
   1. Alteration in Anatomy and Physiology
      a. Decreased sweat glands
      b. Decreased production of melanin and hair follicles
      c. Decreased blood supply to the nail beds
      d. Decreased subcutaneous fat
   2. Assessment
      a. Decreased ability to determine the differences between hot and cold
      b. Lack of skin turgor

      c. Dry hair, grayness, alopecia
      d. Brittle and dull fingernails and toenails
      e. Delayed wound healing
   3. Diagnostic Tests
      a. Blanching sign
      b. Measurement of skin circumference
      c. Measurement of body weight
   4. Nursing Interventions
      a. Instruct the client that she may be unable to distinguish between hot and cold temperatures, providing gloves and blankets for warmth, and use extreme caution when using a heating pad.
      b. Encourage an adequate intake of fluids to enhance skin turgor.
      c. Encourage an adequate intake of protein to enhance wound healing.
      d. Instruct the client to lubricate the skin daily.
      e. Instruct the client to bathe less frequently.
      f. Inform the client to provide adequate humidity in the environment.
H. Genitourinary System
   1. Alterations in Anatomy and Physiology
      a. Decreased size of the kidney
      b. Decreased renal blood flow
      c. Weak bladder and pelvic muscles
      d. Decreased number of nephrons
      e. Decreased glomerular filtration rate
   2. Assessment
      a. Inability to concentrate urine, resulting in dilute urine
      b. Urinary frequency, urgency, nocturia, retention, and incontinence
      c. Enlarged prostate in male clients
      d. Increased incidence of urinary tract infection
   3. Diagnostic Tests
      a. Genitourinary examination
      b. Renal scan
      c. Kidney, ureter, and bladder x-ray
   4. Nursing Interventions
      a. Instruct the client on an adequate oral intake.
      b. Maintain an accurate intake and output.
      c. Encourage the client to go to the bathroom every 2–3 hours.
      d. Avoid catheterization because that increases the incidence of urinary infections.
      e. Instruct the client to avoid fluids and caffeine at bedtime
I. Reproductive System
   1. Alterations in Anatomy and Physiology
      a. Decreased levels of estrogen in the female client
      b. Sclerotic penile veins and arteries

2. Assessment
   a. Decreased production of vaginal secretions
   b. Painful intercourse
   c. Decreased ability to produce an erection
   d. Less frequency of ejaculations
3. Diagnostic Tests: Examination of the genital system
4. Nursing Interventions
   a. Instruct the client on good perineal care.
   b. Instruct the client to use vaginal lubricant for vaginal dryness and painful intercourse.
   c. Explore alterations to sexual activity such as rest before and after sexual activity.

◼ RELATED ISSUES OCCURRING WITH AGING

A. Sleep and Rest
   1. Alterations in sleep and rest
      a. Older adults spend less time in REM and Stage 4 sleep.
      b. Older adults may need only 6-7 hours of sleep a night and a nap in the Afternoon, or they may stay up much later than they did when younger and sleep later in the morning.
      c. The ability to have quality sleep and rest is contingent on getting enough exercise and activity during waking hours.
   2. Assessment
      a. The presence of comorbid conditions may influence the quality and quantity of rest and sleep such as:
         1) Pain
         2) Depression
         3) Immobility
         4) Medications that cause insomnia such as bronchodilators (theophylline, aminophylline), stimulants (caffeine, atropine), or selective serotonin reuptake inhibitors if taken at night
         5) Medications that interfere with REM sleep such as some sleeping preparations
         6) Illicit drugs (amphetamines) and alcohol consumption
         7) Dementia with agitation and wandering
         8) Sleep apnea
         9) Anxiety
         10) Incontinence
   3. Diagnostic Tests
      a. Sleep studies
      b. Levels of stimulants such as theophilline
      c. Evaluation of thyroid function

NURSING ALERT

You need to provide rest periods for geriatric clients in the hospital setting.

4. Nursing Interventions
   a. Observe the client's rest and sleep periods.
   b. Monitor oxygen saturation during sleep periods.
   c. Assess pain and client satisfaction with pain management.
   d. Evaluate the effects and adverse reactions of prescribed and OTC drugs.
   e. Question the client if she self-medicates with alcohol or drugs, attempting to increase sleep or rest.
   f. Formulate a schedule for rest and sleep periods with the client.
   g. Implement methods of promoting sleep and rest such as adequate daytime activity, developing a bedtime routine, a fan or white noise machine to overcome background noises, toileting before bedtime, a warm bath in the evening, massage, bedtime snack or warm milk, decreased fluids after 6 p.m. to prevent awakening to go to the toilet, and no caffeine after 4 p.m.
   h. Instruct the client to use a night-light. In addition to providing a lighted path when the client gets out of bed, a night-light will also prevent shadows in the room which may be confused for people or objects.
   i. Avoid using side rails. Use a very low bed with a bedside floor pad if the client has nighttime confusion to prevent falls or injury.
   j. Encourage the client to continue with previous nighttime routines such as using small amounts of alcoholic beverages to promote sleep if not contraindicated.
   k. Monitor the client for paradoxical effects of prescribed or OTC sleeping medications that may lead to agitation, confusion and insomnia. If REM sleep is interrupted or decreased, the client may be confused or delirious. This may be mistaken for dementia.
B. Immunity
   1. Alterations in Immunity
      a. Immunity in the older adult decreases with a decreased protein and is a major factor.
      b. Lymphocyte production is directly related to protein intake.
      c. If serum albumin is low then the lymphocyte count will be correspondingly low.

NURSING ALERT

A sking a geriatric client for a 24-hour recall of their diet is a useful tool in assessing the client's diet.

2. Assessment
   a. Malnutrition
   b. Delayed wound healing
   c. Comorbid conditions or medications may also contribute to impaired immunity such as:.
      1) prednisone or prednisolone administration
      2) diabetes mellitus
      3) stress (such as from compounded losses—spouse, job, health, home).
      4) HIV
3. Diagnostic Tests
   a. Complete white count with differential
   b. Serum antibody levels
4. Nursing Interventions
   a. Assess the amount of protein the client eats, understanding that older adults often do not eat enough protein because of cost, lack of interest in cooking, or inability to chew food.
   b. Assess the client for infections such as fungus in the mouth, vagina, perianal area; virus such as herpes simplex I and II, herpes zoster as shingles; respiratory infections; bacteria such as pneumonia, bladder, and wound infections.
   c. Monitor vital signs.
   d. Inspect the skin frequently.
   e. Assess the client for confusion because this may be the first indication of infection, especially in the lungs or bladder.
   f. Monitor lung sounds.
   g. Monitor laboratory data related to immune function such as white count (without enough ingested protein, the white count may not be elevated in the presence of a bacterial infection).
   h. Administer supplemental dietary protein to alleviate low serum albumin.
   i. Prevent infection with adequate nutrition, appropriate immunizations for age such as influenza, pneumonia, tetanus, and diphtheria.
   j. Encourage the client to eat adequate protein, change positions frequently, exercise, and increase fluids to prevent skin breakdown and promote healthy skin.

CLIENT TEACHING CHECKLIST

A dequate protein intake may be encouraged by educating clients on food high in protein that may be easier to prepare and digest than traditional meat protein, including:

- Baked beans
- Tofu
- Milk
- Cheese
- Soy milk

C. Nutrition
   1. Alterations in Nutrition
     a. Significant changes in the gastrointestinal tract
     b. Dentition may change with the loss of teeth and the presence of gingivitis.
     c. Gastrointestinal motility and stomach emptying may slow.
     d. Gastric acidity and reflux may increase.
     e. Intestinal motility and absorption of nutrients may decrease.
     f. Metabolism is slower.
     g. Changes in taste and smell may decrease appetite.
   2. Assessment
     a. Decreased appetite
     b. Difficulty chewing
     c. There may be comorbid conditions which affect nutrition such as:
       1) Diabetes mellitus
       2) Pernicious anemia
       3) Difficulty swallowing
       4) Dementia
       5) Decreased activity and mobility
       6) Polypharmacy that may decrease appetite; drug interactions, drug-food interactions.
       7) Hyper- or Hypothyroidism
       8) Malignancy
   3. Diagnostic Tests
     a. Upper and lower GI studies
     b. Dental examination
     c. Swallowing study
     d. Serum levels of vitamin B_{12}, iron, folic acid, and ferritin.

4. Nursing Interventions
   a. Obtain a written 24-hour dietary recall by the client.
   b. Perform a physical assessment of the mouth, hair, GI function, skin, elimination patterns.
   c. Obtain an accurate weight.
   d. Assess the basal metabolic rate.
   e. Assess the client's ability to chew.
   f. Assess mental status, access to food, ability to prepare food, ability to purchase food, home arrangement, and safety with food storage and preparation.
   g. Identify all prescribed medications, OTC, herbal supplements, home remedies, vitamins, and dietary enhancements the client uses. Generally, fiber, medications, and alcohol will decrease appetite. The one exception is marijuana, which will increase the appetite.
   h. Monitor the older adult to determine:
      1) Carbohydrate intake: should be 50–60% of daily calories
      2) Protein intake: should be 10–20%
      3) Fat intake: should be less than 30% of daily calories unless prescribed otherwise
      4) Water soluble vitamins: vitamins B and C will be lost in the urine if the client is taking a diuretic or is losing excessive water in the urine from hyperglycemia.
      5) Fat-soluble vitamins: vitamins A, D, E, K will not be absorbed from the GI tract if the client is taking oil-containing laxatives, such as mineral oil, or is on a very low-fat diet.
   i. Assess the client's appetite (small amounts of beer or red wine with or before meals may stimulate the appetite of the older adult).
   j. Assess for possible older adult abuse or neglect in regard to withholding funds or nutrition.
   k. Plan exercise daily within the client's limitations and abilities (walking for 30 minutes per day is often the best exercise).
   l. Provide nutrient-dense foods which can be chewed and swallowed easily. If dysphagia is present, liquids will need to be thickened to facilitate safe swallowing and prevent aspiration.
   m. Provide a social atmosphere where the older adult does not have to eat alone and will not be rushed.
   n. Provide utensils which the client can easily use such as straws, or large-handled silverware.
   o. Feed the client only if she cannot feed herself so autonomy, rather than learned helplessness, can be fostered.

p. Promote adequate nutrition by providing balanced meals with fiber (such as bran and psyllium), vitamins, minerals (including calcium with vitamins because the older adult often is not in the sunshine enough to make her own vitamin D).

q. Offer finger foods that are easily chewed and swallowed for the client with dementia and agitation.

r. Offer frequent nutritious snacks. Older adults tend not to eat adequate meals.

s. Instruct the client how to increase the most often decreased nutrients (protein and calcium).
   1) Increase protein in the diet by including ground meats, dairy products, adding nonfat dry milk to foods such as milk shakes, meatloaf, and scrambled eggs. Add egg whites to meatballs, hamburgers, casseroles, and baked goods.
   2) Increase calcium intake to 1,200–1,500 mg a day through OTC supplements with vitamin D and dairy products.

t. Increase fluids to 2,000 ml a day. Older adults often do not drink enough fluids to avoid frequent trips to the toilet.

u. Evaluate appropriateness of restricted diets. Does not adding table salt to food decrease the taste so that the client does not eat? Does decreasing the percentage of ingested calories from fat to below 30% affect the absorption of fat-soluble vitamins vitamins A, D, E,K) as well as the taste of foods? Does decreasing fat lead to decreasing protein intake? Does decreasing the intake of calcium by decreasing dairy products?

v. Discuss with the client or family the necessity of a feeding tube if oral intake declines severely. Encourage the family to determine what the client would prefer if there are no advance directives. Support the decision of the family.

D. Pain
   1. Alterations in Pain
      a. Older adults often are unwilling to "complain" and talk about their pain.
      b. Older adults may think that pain is an inevitable part of aging, which it is not.

NURSING ALERT

Religious and cultural beliefs may keep the geriatric client from reporting pain.

    c. Older adults may not want to ask for pain medication because they do not want to "bother" the caregiver.

    d. Older adults may decline pain medications because they are afraid of becoming addicted.

    e. Pain may be viewed as a part of life which must be tolerated or as a punishment for transgressions in life.

2. Assessment
    a. Crying
    b. Rubbing a body part
    c. Moaning
    d. Depression

3. Nursing Interventions
    a. Assess the client's behavior and activity. Watch for decreased activity, insomnia, and restlessness.
    b. Utilize a visual pain scale that the older adult can see and understand easily.
    c. Administer the lowest possible dose of a drug, titrating the drug upward until the level of pain control is acceptable to the client.
    d. Administer drugs to the older adult in the IV or oral routes. The absorption of IM medications is unpredictable in the older adult.
    e. Assess the level of sedation and respiratory rate frequently.
        1) Respiratory depression is more likely with the first dose of an opioid, rather than later doses.
        2) Use adjuvant drugs such as NSAIDs and tricyclic antidepressants to support opioids.
        3) Round-the-clock dosing is the method of choice.
        4) Morphine is the opioid of choice for severe pain.
        5) Assess for GI distress or bleeding, or both, if the older adult is using NSAIDs for pain relief.
        6) Chronic pain may result in depression and spiritual distress.
        7) Every older adult who is taking opioids for pain must be on a bowel regimen, including dietary fiber, stool softener, adequate fluid intake, and a laxative, if needed.

NURSING ALERT

E ncourage the geriatric client to have all medications filled at the same pharmacy. This intervention will help decrease drug–drug interactions.

    f. Identify what nonpharmacologic methods provide pain relief for the client such as massage, heat or cold application (with caution), hydrotherapy, meditation, guided imagery, relaxation therapy, or prayer.

E. Polypharmacy

    a. Older adults often take many prescribed and OTC medications.

    b. Prescribed medications and OTC medications may interact with each other and with food.

    c. Older adults may not be able to afford all of the prescribed medications.

    d. Older adults may not be able to manage the complexities of multiple drugs at different times of the day.

    e. Visual impairments may affect the safety of self-administrations of the many medications.

    f. Older adults metabolize medications more slowly because of changes in liver and kidney function associated with aging and comorbid conditions.

    g. Malabsorption in the GI tract will slow the absorption of drugs.

    h. The systemic effects of drugs will be affected by alterations in circulation.

    i. Diagnostic Tests

        1) Peaks and troughs of medications

        2) Serum levels of medications

    j. Nursing Interventions

        1) Determine the safety of the client's storage and self-administration of medications.

        2) Identify interactions among prescribed medications, OTC drugs, herbal preparations, and client's diet.

        3) Inform all of the client's physicians of all drugs taken.

        4) Determine if the client actually takes all prescribed medications as directed by counting pills in prescription bottles.

        5) Set up a week's medications in a safety container as prescribed.

        6) Identify interactions and side effects of medications

  a) Do any medications such as antidepressants adversely affect the client's appetite?

  b) Does the sheer size and number of medications such as large calcium, fiber, or potassium pills present a safety risk or decrease appetite?

  c) Is the client's quality of life affected by the medication schedule or financial burden?

  d) Instruct the client and family on all medications, interactions, and potential adverse reactions

 7) Determine the safest way to administer medications such as crushing, thickening liquids, or a routine schedule.

F. Communication

 1. Speak clearly and in a normal tone of voice until the older adult's hearing ability is determined.

 2. Stand in the client's direct line of vision. Do not approach from behind.

 3. Ask permission to sit near the client or stand close by and touch the client as appropriate.

 4. Identify the client's level of schooling and ability to read. What language does the client speak and read? Provide an interpreter as needed.

 5. Keep instructions simple. Provide instructions in writing as well as verbally.

 6. Speak to the older adult and not "over" or around her.

 7. When interviewing the older adult, keep questions simple. Allow time for a reply. It may take the older adult longer to formulate an answer.

 8. Encourage the family to allow the older adult to talk.

 9. When instructing the older adult about her care or condition, provide information simply, verbally, and in writing, with schedules and directions clearly described.

 10. Acknowledge the whole person, including her culture, ethnicity, and religion.

 11. The older adult has a cultural and an experiential background which influences who she is today and how she will respond to health problems.

 12. The cohort or experiential group to which the client belongs may identify how she handles problems—such as being a World War II veteran, a Vietnam Veteran, or a baby boomer.

 13. Older adults are more different from each other than alike.

 14. Older adults should be treated as unique individuals.

 15. Avoid discrimination based on age, income, culture, race, ethnicity, religion, or choice of lifestyle

REVIEW QUESTIONS

1. A 92-year-old client with emphysema is experiencing chest pain. The nurse determines with a pulse oximetry that the oxygen saturation is 83%. The nurse understands that it is essential that oxygen be administered by nasal cannula at which of the following rates?

    1. 8 L/minute

    2. 2 L/minute

    3. 5 L/minute

    4. 12 L/minute

2. An 86-year-old client has sustained a fractured femur and has had surgery to repair the fracture. The client is rubbing the surgical site and moaning. Which of the following is the priority nursing intervention?

    1. Administer the prescribed pain medication

    2. Assess the client's pain level

    3. Determine when the client last had pain medication

    4. Inspect the surgical site

3. Which of the following is the appropriate assessment for respiratory depression in the older adult after the administration of an opioid for analgesia? Respiratory depression is

    1. more likely after several doses of the same drug.

    2. most likely after the first dose.

    3. unlikely because the opioid is not prescribed for the older adult in large doses.

    4. unlikely if the drug is given orally.

4. A 73-year-old client has just undergone a colostomy for cancer of the colon. The client tells the nurse the pain is "8" on a scale of 0 to 10. Which of the following is the expected outcome of the nursing care for this client?

    1. The client does not ask for pain medication

    2. The client self-medicates with an over-the-counter medication

    3. The client verbalizes satisfaction with the level of pain and pain control

    4. The client states the pain is "4" on a scale of 0 to 10

5. The nurse assesses which of the following physiological manifestations as indicating that the client is experiencing acute pain? Select all that apply:

    [ ] 1. Verbalization of pain

    [ ] 2. Crying

[ ] **3.** Hypertension

[ ] **4.** Flushing

[ ] **5.** Tachycardia

[ ] **6.** Moist skin

6. The nurse assesses a 67-year-old client suspected of having a cataract for which of the following clinical manifestations? Select all that apply:

[ ] **1.** Halos around lights

[ ] **2.** Decrease in vision

[ ] **3.** Eye pain

[ ] **4.** Abnormal color perception

[ ] **5.** Glare

[ ] **6.** Headache

7. The nurse is establishing the goal for the care of a 93-year-old client who experienced a cerebral vascular accident (CVA) two weeks ago and is hospitalized on a rehabilitation unit. What is the appropriate goal associated with rehabilitation? _____

8. The nurse assesses a 92-year-old client who has experienced a recent cerebral vascular accident (CVA) with a cranial nerve VII dysfunction to be exhibiting which of the following manifestations?

1. Loss of sense of smell

2. Ptosis

3. Difficulty in swallowing

4. Asymmetry of facial features

9. A nursing intervention for a healthy older adult includes providing an adequate oral intake of fluids daily. The rationale for this activity is that older adults tend to drink less than a normal fluid intake and are prone to what electrolyte imbalance? _____

10. The nurse should include which of the following foods that has the most potassium per serving when instructing a 72-year-old client about foods that are high in potassium?

1. Milk

2. Oranges

3. Colas

4. Chicken

11. Which of the following is a priority for the nurse to assess when evaluating the hydration of an 87-year-old client?

1. Height and weight
2. Previous 24-hour intake
3. Skin turgor on the back of the hand
4. Blood pressure

12. During physical assessment of an older adult, the nurse should report which of the following cardiovascular changes that has occurred as a result of dehydration?
    1. Widened pulse pressure
    2. Tachycardia
    3. Hypertension
    4. Decreased respiratory rate

13. The nurse evaluates which of the following nursing assessment findings to be consistent with overhydration in a 72-year-old client admitted with congestive heart failure?
    1. Periorbital edema
    2. Edema of the hands
    3. Projectile vomiting
    4. Moist rales

14. An 80-year-old client who is confined to bed because of generalized weakness, confusion, and disorientation is admitted to the hospital with dehydration. The family asks the nurse why the client is being turned every two hours. The nurse responds that turning the client every two hours is necessary to prevent decubitus ulcers as a result of _____ .

15. A 93-year-old client has been functioning independently in the home but has suddenly become confused. A family member asks the nurse, "Does this mean Dad has Alzheimer's disease?" Which of the following is the most appropriate response?
    1. "It is very likely your father has Alzheimer's disease."
    2. "Why do you think your father has dementia?"
    3. "Confusion can be a sign of an infection in an older adult."
    4. "Your father will have to be monitored over time."

16. A member of an older client's family asks the nurse why medications are ordered at half of the usual dose. Which of the following is the most appropriate response?
    1. "Medications for the older adult are prescribed at a pediatric dose."
    2. "The metabolism of the older adult is much like that of a child of the same weight."

3. "Medications for the older adult may be at lower doses initially until responses are evaluated."

4. "Older adults generally take a lower dose of a medication because of the cost."

17. When the nurse is taking a nursing history on a client, the client mentions, "I slipped on a wet spot on the way to the bathroom." Which of the following is a priority for the nurse to ask?

   1. "Have you started on any new medications?"

   2. "Do you drink caffeinated beverages?"

   3. "Have you experienced any incontinent episodes?"

   4. "Have you been feeling excessively weak recently?"

18. Which of the following should the nurse include in the medication instructions for an older adult who has back pain and a mild opioid with codeine has been prescribed?

   1. Assess the respirations three times a day

   2. Increase daily fiber and fluids

   3. Limit the administration of the medication to severe pain

   4. Avoid taking the medication more than two times a day

19. A hospice nurse caring for a terminally ill client should titrate the dose of morphine sulfate given to an older adult based on which of the following assessments?

   1. Blood pressure

   2. Level of consciousness

   3. Level of pain

   4. Request of family

20. An older adult asks the nurse why a daily bath is necessary. The nurse should respond that daily bathing

   1. stimulates circulation, provides relaxation, and mobilizes joints.

   2. adds hydration and prevents dry skin.

   3. including combing and brushing of the hair helps to remove excess oil from the scalp.

   4. is necessary to comply with agency policy.

21. Which of the following should the nurse include in the instructions given to an older adult about self-care and hygiene to achieve a positive outcome?

   1. A detailed description of the procedures

   2. A written description of the outcomes

3. A description of the care center's routines

4. An article on the importance of hygiene

22. The nurse evaluates which factor as a priority that will adversely affect mobility and self-care in the older adult?

1. Weakness

2. Level of consciousness

3. Disease

4. Family assistance

23. Older clients have individual preferences in carrying out activities of daily living (ADLs). The nurse should include which intervention as a priority for encouraging independence in ADLs?

1. Allow the client to decide when to have a bath

2. Ask the client what ADLs are acceptable to perform

3. Provide total care for a client who is handicapped

4. Assess the client's abilities and preferences

24. The nurse finds an 88-year-old client lying on the floor unresponsive. The priority action for the nurse to take is

1. start CPR.

2. notify the physician.

3. place the client back in bed.

4. assess the respirations and pulse.

25. When planning to interview an older adult for a health history, the nurse should consider which of the following as a priority?

1. The purpose of the interview is to obtain pertinent historical data from the client

2. The interview is directed toward offering solutions to the client's problems

3. The interview should be conducted in the client's room

4. The goals of the interview vary

26. The registered nurse is planning clinical assignments for a geriatric nursing unit. Which of the following assignments should the nurse delegate to a licensed practical nurse?

1. Assess a 67-year-old client after cataract surgery

2. Monitor the serum electrolytes in an 87-year-old client with renal failure

3. Take the vital signs of a 71-year-old client following a hip arthroplasty

4. Perform a physical assessment on a 62-year-old client admitted for abdominal pain

ANSWERS AND RATIONALES

1. **2.** In emphysema, the drive to breathe will be decreased or eliminated if oxygen is administered at a high rate. The best and safest initial rate of oxygen flow is 2 L to 3 L/minute. If higher flow rates are administered, the client may need artificial ventilation.

2. **2.** Older adults may rub or pat a painful area rather than verbalize the pain. The priority intervention is to assess the client's pain level by asking the client. Administering pain medications, determining when the client had the last pain medication, and inspecting the surgical site are all appropriate interventions, but only after the current level of pain is assessed.

3. **2.** Depending on the pain level, large doses may be prescribed for older adults. If a client is very sensitive to an opioid, the resulting respiratory depression is most likely to occur after the first dose. The route of administration will not decrease the likelihood of respiratory depression.

4. **3.** An older adult in severe pain may not ask for pain medication because of a reluctance to "complain." The nurse cannot determine for the client what is an acceptable level of pain. A good outcome is achieved when the client can verbalize satisfaction with the level of pain and pain control.

5. **3, 5.** Hypertension and tachycardia are physiological manifestations of acute pain. Crying and verbalizing pain are psychological or emotional manifestations of pain. When a client is in acute pain, the skin is more likely to cool and pale.

6. **2, 4, 5.** A decrease in vision, abnormal color perception, and glare are clinical manifestations with cataracts. Halos around lights are common in glaucoma. Eye pain and headaches may be present in a variety of other eye disorders.

7. **Prevent and treat physical deformities.** Rehabilitation begins when the client enters the health care system. The overall goal of rehabilitation is to prevent and treat physical deformities.

8. **4.** An asymmetry of facial features is specific to cranial nerve VII, the facial nerve. A difficulty in swallowing is associated with cranial nerve IX, the glossopharyngeal nerve. Loss of smell is common with injury to cranial nerve I, the olfactory nerve. Ptosis occurs with damage to the cranial nerve III, the oculomotor nerve.

9. **Hypernatremia.** Older adults are prone to hypernatremia because of hemoconcentration from a decreased intake of fluids. Hyponatremia may occur from fluid overload, decreased sodium intake, or diuretic use.

10. **2.** Citrus fruits, such as oranges, have the highest concentrations of potassium.

11. 4. Although weight and previous intake are important in evaluating hydration, blood pressure will give a more accurate indication of current hydration. Skin turgor should be checked in the older adult on the clavicle or forehead. A 24-hour intake of fluids may provide the nurse with additional information about the client's hydration status, but it is not the priority.

12. 2. A narrowed pulse pressure and hypotension indicate dehydration and decreased circulating blood volume. Tachycardia and an increased respiratory rate indicate the body is attempting to increase the circulation of oxygen in the blood.

13. 4. Periorbital edema and edema of the hands are related to kidney failure and overhydration. Projectile vomiting in the older adult may be related to increased intracranial pressure. Moist rales indicate left-sided heart failure in a client with congestive heart failure.

14. Pressure. Pressure on the tissues and lack of relief from the pressure are the causes of decubiti. Turning the client every two hours alleviates the pressure.

15. 3. An older adult client who suddenly becomes confused may have developed an infection, generally of the lungs and bladder, or may be dehydrated. Confusion that occurs in delirium, Alzheimer's disease, and other forms of dementia develops slowly and over time. Telling a client's family that the client may have dementia and will have to be monitored over time shuts down communication. Telling the family that the acute confusion may be a sign of infection keeps communication open and offers information. Rather than a "why" question, the nurse could ask for more recent history on the client, such as whether the client has experienced a fall or head injury.

16. 3. Older adults do not metabolize medications at the same rates as children and younger adults do. The liver and kidneys may have impaired function. Even though a thin older adult may have a body weight similar to that of a child, the dosage of medications must allow for age and comorbid conditions.

17. 3. Although asking clients if they have started on any new medications, drink caffeinated beverages, or are excessively weak are relevant when taking a health history, the possibility of incontinence is significant since the client stated that the fall was the result of "slipping on a wet spot."

18. 2. It is difficult for clients to count their own respirations accurately, and that measure is not necessary when taking codeine. The dosing of the medication should be "round the clock" to prevent severe pain. Older adult clients are more prone to constipation than younger clients, and fiber and fluids should be increased in the diet.

19. 3. The level of pain acceptable to the client determines the dose of pain medication given to a hospice client. The pain medication is then titrated.

20. 1. Daily bathing may damage fragile skin in the older adult. Daily combing and brushing of the hair helps stimulate the scalp and distribute the oil. Reasons for daily bathing include stimulating circulation, providing relaxation, and mobilizing joints.

21. 2. By giving the client a written description of the expected outcomes and then explaining the procedures and demonstrating the techniques, the nurse will facilitate learning and mutual goal setting.

22. 1. Older adults may have many chronic conditions that do not affect mobility or self-care. Weakness from any cause often means that older adults cannot be mobile and care for themselves.

23. 4. It is not advised to ask older clients when they want to take a bath because they may refuse ADLs. Even clients who are handicapped are capable of autonomy and self-care. Asking the client what ADLs are acceptable to perform promotes dependency. Assessing the client's abilities, setting mutual goals, and planning care accordingly promote independence in the client.

24. 4. When finding a client unresponsive on the floor, the priority is to assess the respirations and pulse before notifying the physician or starting CPR.

25. 4. The interview for a health history should identify past and present problems. It should be conducted in a private environment, and the client's room may not be private. The interview is not for the purpose of offering solutions to the problems. Depending on the setting and the reasons why the nurse is conducting the interview (such as to assess an acutely ill client or to evaluate a client still living at home who has a chronic condition), the goals may vary.

26. 3. A licensed practical nurse may take the vital signs on a client following a hip arthroplasty. Assessing, monitoring, and performing a physical assessment are all skills that require a registered nurse.

Delirium and Dementia

2

◼ DEPRESSION

A. Description

1. Depression is not a normal part of aging and can be initially confused with delirium or dementia.

2. Up to 30% of older women and 20% of older men may have clinical depression.
3. Depression is undertreated in the older adult and can lead to a diminished quality of life and increased risk of suicide.
4. The depression may be linked to a significant loss or life change.
5. Older adults who are at great risk for suicide are single men without a close support system who have chronic illnesses, chronic pain, or a terminal illness.
6. The client may-self medicate with alcohol or other drugs for the depression.
7. Denial, rationalization, and projection are often the coping mechanisms which prevent the client and family from seeking professional help.
8. Depression is generally diurnal, with clinical manifestations worse in the morning.
9. Generally, depression has persisted longer than 2 weeks and may last for years.

B. Assessment

1. Clinical manifestations of depression in the older adult may be typical or atypical.
2. Anorexia or overeating, especially sweets and starches
3. Angry outbursts
4. Forgetfulness or decreased attention span
5. Insomnia or sleeping too much
6. Loss of interest in hygiene, previous activities, or the future
7. Delusions and paranoia
8. Substance abuse (alcohol and drugs)
9. Psychomotor retardation or agitation
10. Apathy
11. Restless sleep with early morning awakening
12. May be at risk for suicide

NURSING ALERT

G eriatric clients may not relate to the term "depression," but may better relate to terms such as feeling "blue" or "down."

DELEGATION TIP

R N$_s$ need to advise assistive personnel to inform them if there are changes in a geriatric client's appetite, sleeping patterns, hygiene habits, or behavior. These may be indicative of depression.

C. **Nursing Diagnosis**
   1. Adult Failure to thrive
   2. Chronic confusion
   3. Disturbed thought processes
D. **Diagnostic tests**
   1. Geriatric Depression Scale
   2. Beck Depression Inventory Scale
   3. Center for Epidemiological Studies—Depression Scale
   4. Medical examination with laboratory testing to rule out central nervous system infection such as syphilis or HIV
E. **Nursing Interventions**
   1. Assess for clinical manifestation of depression after significant life events such as a loss of a spouse or close relative, a job, health, or a move
   2. Assess changes in appearance, weight, sleep patterns, affect, and ability to function.
   3. Monitor the client for verbalization of hopelessness, fear of the future, crying, loss of interest in prized possessions, relationships, and self-care.
   4. Discuss depression and the client's feelings.
   5. Refer for neuropsychiatric evaluation, medication, and psychotherapy as appropriate.
   6. Monitor a client taking antidepressants for adverse reactions such as agitation, insomnia, anorexia and weight loss.
   7. Encourage the client to write feelings in a journal.
   8. Utilize planned reminiscence therapy to emphasize life accomplishments whether in a group or individually.
   9. Monitor for possible self-directed harm: report and refer as warranted; remove items that could be used for self-harm such as cords, plastic bags, firearms, knives drugs, and institute suicide precautions.

NURSING ALERT

W hen a client is admitted with a decrease in cognitive function, it is very important for you to discern over what period of time the change has occurred. If the change has occurred rapidly, medical causes should be explored immediately.

10. Contract with the client that he will not harm himself or others.
11. Identify contribution of losses to depression and help client handle these losses.

■ DELIRIUM

A. **Description**
   1. A decrease in cognitive function and possible alteration in consciousness which is reversible
   2. The cognitive changes occur rapidly, such as in a few hours or within a day, and a cause can usually be determined and often corrected.
   3. Common causes:
      a. Hypernatremia
      b. Hyponatremia
      c. Dehydration
      d. Fever greater than 104°F or 40°C
      e. Medication adverse reactions or interactions
      f. Low blood glucose
      g. Ketoacidosis
      h. Hypoxia
      i. Concussion
      j. Increased intracranial pressure from traumatic brain injury
      k. Subdural hematoma
      l. Drug or alcohol abuse
      m. Sensory overload or deprivation
      n. Sleep deprivation
   4. Rapid onset often being worse at night
B. **Assessment**
   1. Fluctuation awareness and orientation
   2. Disorganized thinking
   3. May experience illusions, delusions, or hallucinations
   4. Hypokinetic or hyperkinetic
   5. Sleeplessness, with the cycle often reversed
   6. Clinical manifestations, often worse at night
C. **Nursing Diagnosis**
   1. Adult Failure to thrive
   2. Acute confusion
   3. Disorganized thought processes

D. Diagnostic Tests

1. Diagnostic testing may be used to confirm a cause of the delirium or to rule out a cause, such as a CT of the head to rule out trauma or bleeding.
2. Serum electrolyte, complete blood counts, blood sugars, and drug screens
3. Urinalysis and chest x-ray are necessary to indicate the presence of infection.
4. An ECG and serial enzyme levels may be used to determine cardiac causes.
5. Oxygenation saturation levels

E. Nursing Interventions

1. Assess and carefully document level of consciousness and changes in mental status.
2. Monitor oxygen saturation and laboratory tests.
3. Protect from injury. Institute safe measures such as side rails up, not leaving the client alone, and seizure precautions.
4. Correct the underlying cause of delirium such as administering oxygen, feeding the client in the presence of low blood sugar, rehydrating if there is dehydration, promoting restful sleep, or administering antibiotics.
5. Reorient to person, place, and time as indicated.
6. Make sure a client who wear eyeglasses or uses a hearing aid has them on.
7. Avoid the use of restraints.
8. Monitor the client for complications of immobility, and implement activities such as range of motions to prevent skin breakdown.
9. Offer support to the client and family.
10. Administer antipsychotics such as haloperidol (Haldol), risperidone (Risperdal), quetiapine (Seroquel), and olanzapine (Zyprexa). See Chapter 28 on Antipsychotics.

■ DEMENTIA/ALZHEIMER'S DISEASE

A. Description

1. A slow loss of cognitive function, with the major sign initially being short-term memory loss.
2. Progresses to death, often without a definitive cause being diagnosed
3. Occurs most often in the older adult but can occur in a younger client with brain injury or Down syndrome
4. There are many known causes of dementia such as neurodegenerative, vascular, metabolic, immunologic, systemic, trauma, or drugs.
5. Many dementias are often mistakenly called "Alzheimer's."
6. If all other possible causes of dementia have been ruled out, a client will be diagnosed with Alzheimer's-like dementia (ALD).

CLIENT TEACHING

The educational needs of caregivers of clients with Alzheimer's include:

- What to expect in each stage of the disease
- Techniques to decrease agitation
- Safety measures

TABLE 2-1   Stages of Alzheimer's Disease

Stage	Clinical Manifestations
Stage 1: Early	Forgetfulness, often subtle and masked by the client
	Indecisiveness
	Increasing self-centeredness; decreasing interest in others, environment, social activities
	Difficulty in learning new information
	Slowed reaction time
	Beginnings of compromised performance at home and at work
Stage 2: Middle	Progressing forgetfulness, inability to remember names of family members or close friends
	Tendency to lose things
	Confusion
	Fearfulness
	Easily induced frustration and irritability; sometimes, angry outbursts
	Repetitive storytelling
	Beginnings of communication problems (inability to remember words, apparent aphasia)
	Inability to follow simple directions
	Difficulty in calculating numbers
	Beginnings of getting lost in familiar places
	Evasive or anxious interactions with others
	Physical activity (pacing, wandering)
	Changes in sleep–rest cycle (with frequent activity at night)

Continued

Table 2-1 Continued

Stage	Clinical Manifestations
	Changes in eating patterns (possible constant hunger or none at all)
	Neglect of ADL and personal hygiene; changes in bowel and bladder continence; and dressing difficulties
	Inability to maintain safety without supervision
	Losses of social behaviors
	Paranoia
Stage 3: Late	Inability to communicate
	Inability to eat
	Incontinence (urine and feces)
	Inability to recognize family or friends
	Confinement to bed
	Total dependence relative to care

7. Types of dementia include Alzheimer's (plaques and tangles in the brain), vascular or multi-infarct dementia (diminished circulation to multiple small areas of the brain), and brain damage from trauma or infection.
8. Alzheimer's and Alzheimer's-like dementia have a predictable downward trajectory and expected stages (see Table 2-1).

B. Assessment
1. Onset is generally insidious.
2. Progressive clinical manifestations that may be stable over a period of time such as months or years
3. Disoriented to person, place, and time
4. Impaired judgment and abstract reasoning
5. May have illusions, delusions, or hallucinations
6. Sleeplessness with frequent awakenings
7. Difficulty in carrying on a conversation with a difficulty in finding the words

C. Nursing Diagnoses
1. Disturbed Thought Processes
2. Self-Care Deficit
3. Ineffective Coping
4. Wandering
5. Social Isolation
6. Ineffective Therapeutic Regimen Management
7. Ineffective Health Maintenance

DELEGATION TIP

W hen delegating activities of daily living, such as personal hygiene and assisting with meals, in clients with Alzheimer's disease, stressing the importance of maintaining a routine to the assistive personnel is vital.

---

   8. Anxiety
   9. Caregiver Role Strain
D. Diagnostic Tests
   1. Alzheimer's Disease can only be confirmed on autopsy when plaques and tangles are found in the brain.
   2. CT scan and MRI may demonstrate brain atrophy or in late stage, enlarged ventricles, or a decreased size of the brain.
   3. Single-photon emission computed tomography (SPECT), magnetic resonance spectoscopy (MRS), and positron emission tomography (PET) may detect changes early in the disease and monitor treatment response.
   4. Apolipoprotein E 4 (*ApoE4*) is a gene present on chromosome 19 which correlates with and increases the risk of developing Alzheimer's disease.
   5. Mini-mental State Exam assesses the degree of cognitive impairment. The client must be able to read, write, and see to complete the exam.
   6. A urine test measuring isoprostanes (by-products of fat metabolism associated with free radicals) may measure the risk of developing Alzheimer's.
E. Nursing Interventions
   1. Maintain a safe and secure environment at all times.
   2. With early cognitive loss, instruct the client and family on memory tips such as a daily schedule and routine, sticky notes as reminders, household items labeled such as Bob's bathroom or Bob's clothes.
   3. Minimize change in the environment.
   4. Client should carry personal identification at all times, including name, address, phone number, statement of medical condition, and how to contact a family member.
   5. Inform the family about dementia and the expected downward course of the illness.
   6. Provide support for planning long-term care and health care directives.
   7. Administer prescribed medications (see Table 2-2)
   8. Instruct the client and family as appropriate about dementia and how to cope with declining cognitive function.
   9. Prevent family role strain and burnout as much as possible through respite care, support groups, and long-term care when needed.

TABLE 2-2   Drugs Used to Treat Decreased Memory and Cognition in Alzheimer's Disease

Name	Classification	Action	Adverse Reactions	Nursing Interventions
donepezil (Aricept)	Autonomic nervous system agent: cholinesterase inhibitor	Thought to increase acetylcholine in cerebral cortex	Headache, insomnia, fatigue, nausea, vomiting, diarrhea, bradycardia	Monitor for improvement of cognition. monitor for signs and symptoms of GI upset or bleeding. monitor asthma or COPD carefully. monitor for bradycardia and fainting.
rivastigmine (Exelon)	Autonomic nervous system agent: cholinesterase inhibitor	Inhibits acetylcholinesterase in the brain	Asthenia, sweating, syncope, fatigue, malaise, flulike symptoms, nausea, vomiting, diarrhea, anorexia, abdominal pain, dizziness, headache, hyperglycemia	Monitor cognitive function, dizziness, lab test results, weight, anorexia.

galantamine (Reminyl)	Autonomic nervous system agent: cholinergic; cholinesterase inhibitor	Acetylcholinesterase inhibitor	Weight loss, bradycardia, syncope, depression, insomnia, nausea, vomiting, diarrhea	Monitor all systems for significant changes.
tacrine (Cognex)	Autonomic nervous system agent: cholinesterase	Increases acetylcholine in the cerebral cortex	Diaphoresis, agitation, dizziness, confusion, nausea, vomiting, diarrhea, purpura	Monitor all systems for significant changes.

NURSING ALERT

Y ou can identify caregivers that are experiencing role strain. Encouragement from you for the client to receive respite care may decrease or eliminate guilt from the caregiver.

10. Be alert for signs of older adult/client abuse of caregivers or caregiver abuse of the vulnerable client.
11. Avoid saying "Don't you remember when?"
12. Frequent and insistent reminders about the date or current situation such as the death of a spouse may increase the client's agitation.
13. Redirect the client as the best way to handle agitation.
14. Permit wandering within a safe environment.
15. Provide finger foods and drinks to prevent weight loss from the energy expenditure.
16. Implement stop signs on exterior doors or paths on the floor marked with wide tape that may prevent the client from going outside.
17. Use chemical restraint with drugs such as haloperidol (Haldol) or sedatives after other interventions have failed.
18. Assess the client's mental status by asking the client to draw a clock. This brief exam of mental status may indicate the ability to follow directions and the memory of what a clock looks like.
19. Assess weight and changes, appetite, presence of agitation, safety concerns such as wandering, sleeping patterns, and coping by the client and family, and implement interventions as appropriate.
20. Provide a quiet, calm environment for the physical and mental status exam. If the client is agitated or anxious, a trusted significant other should be present. Instruct the family member not to answer for or coach the client.
21. Speak slowly and in short sentences. Express only one idea or question at a time.
22. Approach the client from the front and never from behind. Touch the client by permission only unless it is an emergency.
23. Do not contradict or argue with the client or allow the family to do so. Never utilize questions that begin with "Do you remember when . . . ?"
24. Encourage the client to participate in a positive manner. Keep instructions simple.
25. Utilize an adult day care center as appropriate

REVIEW QUESTIONS

1. The nurse has determined that a confused older adult client who keeps pulling out the intravenous line and indwelling catheter is in need of soft wrist restraints. Which of the following should the nurse include in this client's plan of care?

    1. Obtain a p.r.n. restraint order

    2. Assess the placement of the wrist restraints, skin, and circulation every hour and document

    3. Place the client in a supine position after applying the restraints and secure the wrist restraints to the side rails when the client is in bed

    4. Remove the restraints once every four hours to perform activities of daily living

2. A family expresses concern to the nurse when their 96-year-old mother with dementia living in a long-term care facility seems more confused and does not remember the activities of daily living. Which of the following is the most appropriate response?

    1. "Don't worry, your mother is safe in the long-term care facility."

    2. "You need to remind your mother how to perform her basic needs."

    3. "Your mother will get worse as time goes on and the dementia progresses."

    4. "This must be frustrating for you."

3. A 77-year-old client expresses concern to a nurse in a walk-in psychiatric clinic of "going crazy or of having Alzheimer's disease" because of feelings of being overwhelmed and sad all of the time, and misplacing things. Which of the following is the priority for the nurse to include in this client's plan of care?

    1. Assist the client to develop areas of strength in coping

    2. Make a psychosocial assessment

    3. Explore the available supports for the client

    4. Assure the client and dispel the idea of "going crazy"

4. Upon admission to a long-term care facility, an 83-year-old client is withdrawn, sitting quietly in a chair with the back to the door of the room. When the nurse speaks to the client, the client says, "Go away and leave me alone. Spend your time on someone who can use it. I just don't want to live if I have to stay here." Which of the following is the priority nursing action?

    1. Create a welcoming and cheerful atmosphere

    2. Encourage the client to discuss the feelings of hopelessness

3. Allow the client to have periods of solitude as asked for

4. Assess for depression and suicide potential

5. An 86-year-old client suddenly becomes confused about time, place, and person. After evaluating the oxygen saturation to be 98%, which of the following should the nurse assess first?

1. What medications the client is taking

2. Vital signs

3. Possibility of a recent fall

4. The client's pain level

6. A 56-year-old client diagnosed with Stage I (early-onset) Alzheimer's disease lives at home with family. A daughter asks the nurse, "How long will Dad be like this before his memory returns?" The best initial response the nurse can make is

1. "He may never get better."

2. "This is just the beginning of a predicted decline."

3. "Tell me what you know about Alzheimer's disease."

4. "Is he taking his medicine for Alzheimer's disease?"

7. An older adult is picking at clothing and muttering, "Butterflies are all over me." The nurse does not see any butterflies. Which of the following is the priority for the nurse to perform?

1. Identify any risk for injury related to altered thought processes

2. Call for help

3. Provide a nonstimulating environment

4. Inform the client there are no butterflies in the room

8. An older adult's cognitive function has declined over the last two years. The family is concerned by the loss of short-term memory and the safety issues posed by the forgetfulness. A complete medical workup including a CT scan of the head has shown no medical cause for the cognitive changes. The nurse explains to the client and family that the medical diagnosis of Alzheimer's disease is based on

1. the information that no other cause can be found for the changes.

2. a blood test for C-reactive protein that was positive.

3. a loss of function seen on the Mini-Mental State Exam.

4. the results of an x-ray of the skull showing a decrease in the size of the brain.

9. When assessing an older adult, the nurse should be alert to the clinical manifestations of depression that may be masked by other chronic conditions. The cardinal and primary behavior exhibited in the depressed older adult is

1. a loss of interest in previously pleasurable activities.
2. inactivity.
3. drinking alcohol.
4. crying.

10. Donepezil hydrochloride (Aricept) has been prescribed for a client with Alzheimer's disease. Which of the following adverse reactions should the nurse include in the medication instructions given to the family? Select all that apply:

[ ] 1. Headache

[ ] 2. Tachycardia

[ ] 3. Insomnia

[ ] 4. Hypotension

[ ] 5. Constipation

[ ] 6. Anorexia

11. Before preparing to use the Mini-Mental State Exam for cognitive function in an older adult, the nurse should consider which of the following limitations of the exam?

1. The test takes one hour to administer
2. The client must be able to see and write
3. The exam must take place in a dimly lit room
4. The exam is valid only with English-speaking clients

12. The nurse should consider which of the following medical etiologies in an older adult who has been healthy until recently but has developed dementia?

1. Sexually transmitted diseases
2. Electrolyte imbalances
3. Arthritis
4. Liver disease

13. Which of the following four older adult clients that the nurse is caring for does the nurse evaluate as most at risk for self-directed violence?

1. A 76-year-old single man who lives in a retirement center and engages in community activities
2. A widowed man who is 88 years old, lives alone, and has multiple chronic illnesses
3. An 83-year-old woman who has type 2 diabetes mellitus and lives with her daughter
4. A recently widowed woman with multiple chronic illnesses who lives near family

14. An older adult client with chronic depression tells the nurse, "Don't worry about me. I can manage the pain of my arthritis. The way I mix up my medications helps." The best initial response by the nurse is

    1. "Don't mix your medications yourself. Take them only as prescribed."
    2. "That's dangerous. I'll have to take your narcotics from you."
    3. "That's dangerous. I'll have to call your daughter and have her give you your medications."
    4. "Tell me what you take and how you mix them."

15. The nurse is caring for an older adult with situational depression following the death of a spouse. What is the most important outcome for the nurse to plan for?

    1. The client will discuss the spouse and the meaning of the loss
    2. The client will not cry
    3. The client will speak of the spouse only positively
    4. The client will avoid talking about the spouse and engage in social activities

16. Which of the following is the priority nursing intervention for the nurse to include in the plan of care for a client with behavior problems related to dementia?

    1. Inform the client why the nursing interventions are necessary
    2. Instruct the caregivers on the process of dementia and care to be given
    3. Be consistent by repeating the same intervention as the client's dementia progresses
    4. Assist the client to perform difficult tasks

17. A nurse observes a family member continually reminding a client in late Stage II Alzheimer's disease of the date and place. The client is adamant that it is 1922 and the North Pole. The nurse informs the family member that continually reminding the client of the date and place will result in

    1. a return of memory.
    2. increased retention of the information.
    3. a catastrophic reaction.
    4. an interest in having a calendar.

18. An 80-year-old client is admitted to the intensive care unit because of hemorrhaging after a stent is placed in her left femoral artery to improve circulation to the leg. The client is confused, not following instructions, and pulling at the intravenous tubing and indwelling catheter. The client's adult son tells the nurse, "My mom was never like this before. What have you done to her?" The best initial response the nurse can make is

1. "We've done nothing to her. She must have dementia."

2. "Older adults will become confused after a bleed to the brain from decreased oxygen."

3. "Your mother is acting like she is in alcohol withdrawal. Does she drink?"

4. "You will need to talk to your mother's physician to get information about her condition."

19. An older client in a nursing facility suddenly becomes confused, paranoid, and verbally abusive to the staff. Which of the following is the priority nursing action?

    1. Ask the family members if they had a recent disagreement with the client

    2. Assess the vital signs and obtain a urine specimen

    3. Reorient the client to person, place, and time

    4. Ask whether the client is hearing voices

20. The nurse assesses which of the following behaviors in a client in early Stage I Alzheimer's disease? Select all that apply:

    [ ] 1. Masks forgetful behavior

    [ ] 2. Has a slow reaction time

    [ ] 3. Repetitive storytelling

    [ ] 4. Inability to follow simple directions

    [ ] 5. Becomes angry when challenged

    [ ] 6. Change in eating patterns

21. An older adult client with dementia becomes increasingly confused and wanders away from a long-term facility. The appropriate nursing action is to

    1. call law enforcement officials.

    2. restrain the client.

    3. follow the client and redirect from a safe distance.

    4. offer the client a ride back to the facility.

22. Which of the following should the nurse include in the education provided to a new graduate nurse to protect the nurse from injury when a client with dementia or delirium becomes aggressive?

    1. Gently place a hand on the client's shoulder to promote trust

    2. Lead the client to the activity area where there are others to distract the client

    3. Provide a quiet, calm atmosphere and offer simple directions

    4. Offer the client a meal

23. Donepezil hydrochloride (Aricept) is prescribed for an older adult with early dementia, Alzheimer's-like disease (ALD). When reviewing the client's medical conditions and medications, the nurse notifies the physician that there might be a serious interaction because the client has

    1. osteoarthritis.
    2. cancer of the pancreas.
    3. not had a yearly influenza immunization.
    4. bradycardia.

24. Rivastigmine (Exelon) is prescribed for a client with dementia. Which of the following would be an appropriate outcome of nursing care specific to this drug?

    1. The client will sleep six hours without waking during the night
    2. The client will eat 50% of all meals and snacks
    3. The client will maintain a weight within the normal range
    4. The client will maintain the serum potassium within normal range

25. The nurse assesses that a deficiency in what nutrient places an older adult with dementia at risk for malnutrition? _____

26. The registered nurse is planning the clinical assignments for a geriatric mental health unit. Which of the following assignments should the nurse delegate to a licensed practical nurse?

    1. Develop a plan of care for a client with dementia
    2. Perform a physical assessment on a client with Alzheimer's disease
    3. Administer donepezil hydrochloride (Aricept) to a client newly diagnosed with Alzheimer's disease
    4. Provide education to the family of a client with dementia

ANSWERS AND RATIONALES

1. **2.** The standard of care for restraints is that they can be applied only with a written order from a health care provider. The order must be renewed every 24 hours. A p.r.n. order for restraints is not acceptable. Restraints should be removed once every two hours to perform activities of daily living. The client with wrist restraints should be placed in a lateral position to prevent aspiration. The condition of the skin, circulation, and placement of restraints must be assessed every hour. The assessment must also be documented.

2. **4.** When a family expresses concern over their mother's confusion and decreased ability to perform her activities of daily living, the most

appropriate response to the family is to acknowledge how frustrating it must be for the family. The nurse should not minimize family members' feelings or tell them how to feel. Reminding a client with short-term memory loss may increase agitation. Although the dementia will progress over time, reinforcing that with the family is a negative response and may shut down communication.

3. 2. The first step of the nursing process is assessment. Before helping the client deal with a problem or exploring available resources, the nurse should determine if a problem is really present. Assuring the client and dispelling the idea of "going crazy" are negative interventions, and the nature of this client's condition is not yet known.

4. 4. Although creating a cheerful environment is important in a long-term care facility, the priority intervention is safety. Older adults who express not wanting to live if they have to stay there may be clinically depressed and at risk for self-harm. Encouraging clients to discuss feelings of hopelessness and allowing for periods of solitude may be appropriate interventions, but are not the priorities.

5. 2. In the case of delirium and a sudden change in mental status, the nurse should always assess for physiological causes—airway, breathing, and circulation—first. Although medications the client is taking, a recent fall, or the client's pain level may be possible causes of the delirium, the vital signs should be assessed first.

6. 3. The best response when the family of a client diagnosed with Stage I (early-onset) Alzheimer's disease asks when the family member will get better would be to ask family members how much they know about Alzheimer's. This is the best response because it facilitates open communication. Although the disease has a progressive course, telling the family that will close communication. Asking the family member if the client is taking medication for Alzheimer's disease is an inappropriate response, because it changes the subject.

7. 1. The first nursing action should be to identify any risks to the client or others because of the alteration in thought processes that the client is experiencing. It may be appropriate to provide a nonstimulating environment, but that is not the priority. Informing the client that there are no butterflies might precipitate a catastrophic reaction.

8. 1. The definitive diagnosis for Alzheimer's disease is only found on autopsy. When all other possible causes of cognitive decline are ruled out, the medical diagnosis of Alzheimer's disease (or Alzheimer's-like disease) is made. The Mini-Mental State Exam is one of many short tests to measure cognitive function, but it does not actually diagnose dementia. The older adult will show a decrease in the mass of the brain but may not

have a corresponding loss of cognitive function. A blood test for C-reactive protein would not be positive for Alzheimer's disease.

9. 1. Loss of interest in previously enjoyable activities and withdrawal are indicators to the nurse that the client may be clinically depressed and in need of further assessment. Inactivity, drinking alcohol, and crying may be indicative of depression or other chronic conditions, not just depression.

10. 1, 3, 6. Donepezil hydrochloride (Aricept) is used in the treatment of mild to moderate Alzheimer's disease. Adverse reactions of Aricept include headache, bradycardia, insomnia, hypertension, diarrhea, and anorexia.

11. 2. The Mini-Mental State Exam does not require a specially trained individual and requires only 20 to 30 minutes to administer. The client must be able to see and write because the client will be asked to write a sentence as well as to copy a drawn figure.

12. 1. The first indication that a client has a sexually transmitted disease such as tertiary syphilis or HIV may be cognitive function changes and dementia.

13. 2. Older women, even if depressed, tend to be less likely to harm themselves, because they have social support and other interests. Older men without social support who have multiple chronic illnesses and live alone are more likely to commit suicide than older women.

14. 4. Clients with chronic illnesses and pain often adjust their own medications or add over-the-counter medications. A client's depression could be a result of the drugs or it could be the reason the client mixes medications. The nurse needs further information to identify risks for injury.

15. 1. It is most appropriate for the nurse to encourage clients who are experiencing situational depression over the loss of a spouse to verbalize their feelings. Crying is a normal and healthy expression of loss. The relationship with the spouse may not always have been positive, or the client may feel angry about the death. Setting an outcome that the client will speak positively describes how the client should feel and is not necessarily true.

16. 2. Educating the caregivers, whether family members or others, is always the priority when caring for a client with dementia. The caregivers must understand the disease and expected behaviors as well as the interventions for problem behaviors. The same interventions may not be effective as the condition changes. This should be part of the continued evaluation and part of the replanning.

17. 3. In late Stage II Alzheimer's disease there is no hope for memory return. Repeating reality orientation for the client whose reality is different may

cause anxiety, anger, agitation, and a catastrophic reaction, such as running away or violence.

18. 2. Older adult clients may become confused after a bleed to the brain from decreased oxygen. Telling the family that the medical team has done nothing to the client is a defensive statement and would cut off communication. Dementia is a medical diagnosis, which the nurse does not make. The best initial response by the nurse is to answer the son's question. The nurse may need to know if the client has an alcohol abuse problem, but not until the son's concerns are answered. Passing the son off to the physician at this point would shut down communication with the son.

19. 2. Assessing the vital signs and obtaining a urine specimen is the priority in an older client who suddenly becomes confused and develops psychotic behavior. A urinary tract infection would be evident from an elevated temperature and bacteria in the urine specimen.

20. 1, 2, 5. A client attempts to mask forgetful behavior, has a slow reaction time, and may become angry when challenged in early Stage I Alzheimer's disease. Repetitive storytelling, an inability to follow simple directions, and a change in eating patterns are behaviors exhibited in Stage II Alzheimer's.

21. 3. When a client with dementia wanders away from a long-term care facility, the nurse should see if the client will return willingly with persuasion and redirection. If the client will not return, notifying law enforcement may be necessary, but the presence of law enforcement officials may also agitate and frighten the client. At no time should the nurse physically restrain the client alone or transport a client.

22. 3. Touching an agitated client may increase aggression and precipitate violence against the nurse. The client should be in a quiet, calm atmosphere away from others and simple directions should be offered. Offering a meal may work as a temporary distraction, but the client at this point will be unable to sit and follow instructions about eating.

23. 4. Aricept is a cholinesterase inhibitor used in the treatment of Alzheimer's disease, which may cause bradycardia with fainting.

24. 3. Rivastigmine tartrate is used in the treatment of mild to moderate Alzheimer's disease. Nausea, vomiting, anorexia, and abdominal pain are adverse reactions to Exelon. The nurse should monitor weight weekly. Eating 50% of the food offered may not be sufficient to maintain body weight.

25. Protein. The diets of older adults are often deficient in protein. Protein sources may not be chewable or palatable to the client with dementia. Protein should be added to the diet in the form of protein powder or other easily ingested sources, such as ice cream cones.

26. 3. A licensed practical nurse may administer donepezil hydrochloride (Aricept) to a client with Alzheimer's disease. Developing a plan of care, performing a physical assessment, and providing education to a client's family on dementia are tasks that should be performed by a registered nurse.

Appendices Table of Contents

Appendix A: Review of Systems When Taking a Complete Health History

General

Client's perception of general state of health at the present, difference from usual state, vitality and energy levels

Neurological

Headache, change in balance, incoordination, loss of movement, change in sensory perception/feeling in an extremity, change in speech, change in smell, fainting (syncope), loss of memory, tremors, involuntary movement, loss of consciousness, seizures, weakness, head injury

Psychological

Irritability, nervousness, tension, increased stress, difficulty concentratiing, mood changes, suicidal thoughts, depression.

Skin

Rashes, itching, changes in skin pigmentation, black and blue marks (ecchymoses), change in color or size of mole, sores, lumps, change in skin texture, odors, excessive sweating, acne, loss of hair (alopecia), excessive growth of hair or growth of hair in unusual locations (hirsutism), change in nails, amount of time spent in the sun

Eyes

Blurred vision, visual acuity, glasses, contacts, sensitivity to light (photophobia), excessive tearing, night blindness, double vision (diplopia), drainage, bloodshot eyes, pain, blind spots, flashing lights, halos around objects, glaucoma, cataracts

Ears

Hearing deficits, hearing aid, pain, discharge, lightheadedness (vertigo), ringing in the ears (tinnitus), earaches, infection

Nose and Sinuses

Frequent colds, discharge, itching, hay fever, postnasal drip, stuffiness, sinus pain, polyps, obstruction, nosebleed (epistaxis), change in sense of smell

Mouth

Toothache, tooth abscess, dentures, bleeding/swollen gums, difficulty chewing, sore tongue, change in taste, lesions, change in salivation, bad breath

Throat/Neck

Hoarseness, change in voice, frequent sore throats, difficulty swallowing, pain/ stiffness, enlarged thyroid (goiter)

Respiratory

Shortness of breath (dyspnea), shortness of breath on exertion, phlegm (sputum), cough, sneezing, wheezing, coughing up blood (hemoptysis), frequent upper respiratory tract infections, pneumonia, emphysema, asthma, tuberculosis

Cardiovascular

Shortness of breath that wakes you up in the night (paroxysmal nocturnal dyspnea), chest pain, heart murmur, palpitations, fainting (syncope), sleep on pillows to breathe better (orthopnea; state number of pillows used), swelling (edema), cold hands/feet, leg cramps, myocardial infarction, hypertension, valvular disease, pain in calf when walking (intermittent claudication), varicose veins, inflammation of a vein (thrombophlebitis), blood clot in leg (deep vein thrombosis), anemia

Breasts

Pain, tenderness, discharge, lumps, change in size, dimpling

Gastrointestinal

Change in appetite, nausea, vomiting, diarrhea, constipation, usual bowel habits, black tarry stools (melena), vomiting blood (hematemesis), change in stool color, excessive gas (flatulence), belching, regurgitation, heartburn, difficulty swallowing (dysphagia), abdominal pain, jaundice, hemorrhoids, hepatitis, peptic ulcers, gallstones

Urinary

Change in urine color, voiding habits, painful urination (dysuria), hesitancy, urgency, frequency, excessive urination at night (nocturia), increased urine volume (polyuria), dribbling, loss in force of stream, bedwetting, change in urine volume, incontinence, pain in lower abdomen (suprapubic pain), kidney stones, urinary tract infections

Musculoskeletal

Joint stiffness, muscle pain, back pain, limitation of movement, redness, swelling, weakness, bony deformity, broken bones, dislocations, sprains, gout, arthritis, osteoporosis, herniated disc

Female Reproductive

Vaginal discharge, change in libido, infertility, sterility, pain during intercourse, menses: last menstrual period (LMP), age period started (menarche), regularity, duration, amount of bleeding, premenstrual symptoms, intermenstrual bleeding, painful periods (dysmenorrhea), menopause: age of onset, duration, symptoms, bleeding, obstetrical: number of pregnancies, number of miscarriages/ abortions, number of children, type of delivery, complications, type of birth control, estrogen therapy

Male Reproductive

Change in libido, infertility, sterility, impotence, pain during intercourse, age at onset of puberty, testicular pain, penile discharge, erections, emissions, hernias, enlarged prostate, type of birth control

Nutrition

Present weight, usual weight, food intolerances, food likes/dislikes, where meals are eaten

Endocrine

Bulging eyes, fatigue, change in size of head, hands, or feet, weight change, heat/ cold intolerances, excessive sweating, increased thirst, increased hunger, change in body hair distribution, swelling in the anterior neck, diabetes mellitus

Lymph Nodes

Enlargement, tenderness

Hematological

Easy bruising/bleeding, anemia, sickle cell anemia, blood type

Appendix B: Modifications to Make Based on the Challenging Needs of the Older Adult

1. Flexibility and positional needs	Some older adults may have limited movement and ability to sit up. Obtain assistance or examine in a side-to-side approach. If the older adult is very uncomfortable, delineate only what is important—adventitious breath sounds and abnormalities noted upon inspection and palpation.
2. Cognitive losses beyond normal age-related changes	If the older adult is unable to follow directions (i.e., take a deep breath, cough, etc.), normal inspiration/expiration will have to suffice. Again, differentiate between normal breath sounds and those which are adventitious.
3. Excessive anxiety or emotional dysfunction	Temporarily stop the exam. Spend time on another unrelated activity, preferably one that is soothing. perhaps a break is necessary. Sometimes incorporating the family member or significant other is helpful. However, there may not be one available.

4. **Uninhibited behaviors**

If the older adult does not have a sense of personal privacy, make sure you are in a room where the door can be closed. Also, provide quality examination gowns, which open in the front but which stay closed when necessary. Privacy and dignity have always been emphasized with all patients young and old. It becomes more of an issue when a person is unable to maintain his or her own privacy because of underlying cognitive diseases.

Appendix C: Pressure Ulcer Care by Risk Factors

Risk Factor	Preventive Actions

1. Bed or Chair Confinement	• Inspect skin at least once a day
	• Bathe when needed for comfort or cleanliness.
	• Prevent dry skin.
	• For a person in bed:
	  1. Change position at least every 2 hours.
	  2. Use a special mattress that contains foam, air, gel, or water
	  3. Raise the head of bed as little and for as short a time as possible.
	• For a person in a chair:
	  1. Change position every hour.
	  2. Use foam, gel, or air cushion to relieve pressure
	• Reduce friction by:
	  1. Lifting rather than dragging when repositioning
	  2. Using corn starch on skin.
	• Avoid use of donut-shape cushions.
	• Participate in a rehabilitation program.

2. Inability to Move	• Persons confined to chairs should be repositioned every hour if unable to do so themselves.

Risk Factor	Preventive Actions
	• For a person in a chair who is able to shift his or her own weight, change position at least every 15 minutes. • Use pillows or wedges to keep knees or ankles from touching each other. • When in bed, place pillow under legs from mid-calf to ankle to keep heels off the bed.

3. Loss of Bowel or Bladder Control	• Clean skin as soon as soiled.
	 • Assess and treat urine leaks.
	 • If moisture cannot be controlled:
	   1. Use absorbent pads and/or briefs with a quick-drying surface.
	   2. Protect skin with a cream or ointment.

4. Poor Nutrition	• Eat a balanced diet. • If a normal diet is not possible, talk to health • care provider about nutritional supplements.
5. Lowered Mental Awareness	• Choose preventive actions that apply to the person with lowered mental awareness. For example, if the person is chair-bound, refer to the specific preventive actions outlined in Risk Factor 1.

Appendix D: Laboratory Values in Older Adults

Test	Age-Related Change	Geriatric Value
Hemoglobin	Slightly decreased, related to reduced hematopoiesis	M: 10–17 g/100 ml F: 9–17 g/100 ml
Hematocrit	Slightly decreased, related to reduced hematopoiesis	M: 38%–54% F: 35%–49%
Leukocytes	Decreased, related to decreased T & B lymphocytes	3,100–9,000 cu mm
Sedimentation rate	Slightly increased	Less than 22 mm/hr
Albumin	Decreased, related to reduced liver size and enzyme production	M: 2.3–4.7 g/100 ml F: 2.6–5.0 g/100/ml
Alkaline phosphatase	Increased, related to decreased liver function	M: 21.3–80.8 units F: 19.9–83.4 units
Blood urea nitrogen	Increased, related to compromised renal function	M: 8–35 mg/100 ml F: 6–30 mg/100 ml
Creatinine	Increased	0.4–1.9 mg/100 ml

Test	Age-Related Change	Geriatric Value
Calcium	Slightly decreased	9–10.9 mg/100 ml
Glucose	Increased	140 mg/100 ml
Potassium	Increased	3.0–5.9 MEQ/L
Creatinine clearance	Must be calculated to consider decreased glomerular filtration rate	
Men		(140 − age) × kg body weight divided by 72
Women		(140 − age) × kg body weight × 0.85 divided by 72

Appendix E: Comprehensive Nursing Assessment Checklist to Identify Residents at High Risk for Decreased Fluid Intake

Purpose: to promote hydration, prevent dehydration

Name of resident: _____ Name of nurse: _____

Unit:

Date:

Check off those assessment findings characteristic of the resident. The greater the number of factors or severity of factors, the greater the risk for diminished hydration. Add descriptive clinical comments as needed.

I. Symptoms of dehydration warranting immediate medical and nursing interventions:

—Fever

—Thirst (not a reliable indicator in elders)

—Dry, warm skin

—Dry mucous membranes

—More than one lengthwise division of the tongue (furrowed)

—Decreased urinary output

—Concentrated urine

—Muscular weakness

—Diminished skin turgor *less than usual baseline* (test over sternum or forehead)

—Increased lethargy

—Daily weight loss

—Increased confusion, greater than usual

—Change in baseline mental function

—Constipation

—Sunken eyes (severe dehydration)

—Tachycardia (severe dehydration)

—Hypotension (severe dehydration)

II. Factors associated with hydration problems:

—Age 85 or older

—Physical immobility (cannot get to water, cannot hold cup: assess functional status)

—Current dysphagia; mechanical problems in swallowing

—Cognitive impairment
    A. Unable to request fluids
    B. Unaware of thirst

—Incontinent of urine

—Fluid intake of 1500 ml or less (do not include caffeinated drinks) Attach 2 to 3 days of intake and output:
    A. Day 1
    B. Day 2
    C. Day 3

—Documented impaired oral intake over the past 1 to 2 weeks: Estimated date of onset:

—Currently on intake and output monitoring

—Resident spends most of the day outdoors in dry and hot temperatures 80° F or warmer

—Resident is active or exercises for at least 30 minutes daily or every other day

III. Problems increasing vulnerability
    A. Medical
      —Hypertension

      —Kidney disease

      —Congestive heart failure

      —Any type of dementia

      —Central nervous system disorders

      —Osteoarthritis

      —Osteoporosis

      —Uncontrolled diabetes
    B. Dietary restrictions
      —Fluids

      —Salt

    —Potassium

    —Protein

C. Medications

    —Diuretics   List:

    —Tricyclic antidepressants or lithium   List:

    —Regular use of laxatives   List:

D. Medical history

    —Dehydration

    —Fever

    —Diarrhea/vomiting

    —Infections

    —Difficulty swallowing

E. Immediate return from

    —One day or greater hospitalization

    —Diagnostic testing requiring use of contrast dyes

    —Dental surgery

    —Eye surgery

    —One-day clinic visit

    —Any test requiring administration of nothing by mouth after midnight

IV. Laboratory reports showing *steady increases** in

—Sodium

—Serum blood urea nitrogen

—Creatinine

—Hematocrit

—Serum osmolality

—Urine specific gravity

*Look *for upward changes* in these baseline laboratory values over time; unless the resident is severely dehydrated, these laboratory values may remain within normal limits but will climb slowly as hydration deteriorates

Nurse's signature:

Other pertinent clinical comments by the nurse and the interdisciplinary team followed by signatures:

Appendix F: Physical Signs and Symptoms of Poor Nutritional Status

	Subjective	Objective
1. General appearance	Fatigue, poor sleep, change in weight, frequent infections	Dull affect, apathetic, increased weight, decreased weight
2. Skin	Pruritus, swelling, delayed wound healing	Dry, rough, scaling, flaky, edema, lesions, decreased turgor, changes in color (pallor, jaundice), petechiae, ecchymoses, xanthomas (slightly elevated yellow nodules)
3. Nails	Brittle	Dry, splinter hemorrhages, spoon-shaped, pale
4. Hair	Easily falls out, brittle	Less shiny, dry, changes in color pigment
5. Eyes	Vision changes, night blindness, eye discharge	Hardening and scaling of cornea, conjunctiva pale or red

Continued

	Subjective	Objective
6. Mouth	Mouth sores	Lips: cracked, dry, swollen, fissures around corners Gums: recessed, swollen, bleeding, spongy Tongue: smooth, beefy red, magenta, pale, fissures, sores, increased or decreased in size, increased or decreased papillae Teeth: missing, caries
7. Head and neck	Headaches, decreased hearing	Xanthelasma, irritation and crusting of nares, swollen cheeks (parotid gland enlargement), goiter
8. Heart and peripheral vasculature	Palpitations, swelling	Cardiac enlargement, changes in blood pressure, tachycardia, heart murmur, edema
9. Abdomen	Tender, changes in appetite, nausea, changes in bowel habits	Edema, hepatosplenomegaly
10. Musculoskeletal system	Weakness, pain, cramping, frequent fractures	Muscle tone is decreased, flabby muscles, bowing of lower extremities
11. Neurological system	Irritable, changes in mood, numbness, paresthesia	Slurred speech, unsteady gait, tremors, decreased deep tendon reflexes, loss of position and vibratory sense, paresthesia, decreased coordination

Appendix G: Age-related Skin, Hair, and Nail Changes in Older People

Systemic changes: loss of cells, decreased circulation
- Loss of collagen (**clastosis**) and muscle, thinning, sagging skin, wrinkles
- Decrease in light-touch sensation
- Atrophy of subcutaneous tissue
- Hypertrophy of abdomen, thighs, and upper arms
- Decrease in sweat, **sebum,** and vitamin D production
- Diminished cell replacement
- Diminished response to skin injury

Loss of hair
- Hair thinning, graying
- Pubic, axillary hair thinning
- Decreased growth

Photoaging:
- Due to environmental damage; increases the appearance of "aging"
- Age spots
- Skin tags, benign (**acrochordons**)
- Fine wrinkling; leathery, lax, dry, blotchy skin
- **Telangiectasia** (dilation of small blood vessels, resulting in reddish vascular lesion)
- **Actinic keratoses** (skin tumor)—small scaly patches, pink to reddish
- **Seborrheic keratosis** (benign) epidermal growths

Dry skin: xerosis:
- Decreased moisture of the skin related to decreased **eccrine** (secretes sweat) and **sebaceous** (secretes oils or sebum) **glands**
- Itching (**pruritis**) and inflammation

Nails:
- Thicken, become brittle and hard
- Decrease in growth rate
- Develop longitudinal lines
- Dryness, uneven pigmentation

Adapted from Estes, M. (1998). *Health assessment & physical examination.* Albany: Delmar Publishers.

Appendix H: Types of Edema

Type	Location
Pitting	Edema that is present when an indentation remains on the skin after applying pressure
Nonpitting	Edema that is firm with discoloration or thickening of the skin; results when serum proteins coagulate in tissue spaces
Angioedema	Recurring episodes of noninflammatory swelling of skin, brain, viscera, and mucous membranes; onset may be rapid with resolution requiring hours to days
Dependent	Localized increase of extracellular fluid volume in a depenent limb or area
Inflammatory	Swelling due to an extracellular fluid effusion into the tissue surrounding an area of inflammation
Noninflammatory	Swelling or effusion due to mechanical or other causes not related to congestion or inflammation

Appendix I: Summary of Age-related Vision Changes

Eyes/vision
>   graying of eyebrows and eyelashes
>   atrophy of skin surrounding eyes
>   ↓ corneal sensitivity
>   ↓ corneal reflex
>   tendency for "dry eyes": ↓ tear secretion
>   **arcus senilis:** cloudy ring around the iris
>   ↓ pigment in iris
>   **presbyopia:** ↓ ability to focus, accommodate
>   ↓ lens flexibility, yellowing difficulty discriminating blue-green colors
>   (↓ short wavelength discrimination)
>   ↓ pupillary size and ↓ response to light/dark
>   ↓ tolerance to glare some ↓ in peripheral vision

■ SUMMARY OF AGE-RELATED HEARING CHANGES

Ears/hearing
>   atrophy of external ears, wrinkling dryness and itching of external ears
>   coarser ear hair
>   hardening of **cerume** (ear wax)
>   thickening of eardrum
>   ↓ equilibrium due to vestibular changes
>   **presbycusis:** ↓ hearing acuity
>   - difficulty hearing high frequencies
>   - difficulty tolerating loud noises and background noises
>   - symptoms are bilateral ↓ ability to discern consonants ("g", "s", "f", etc. create high-frequency sounds)

Appendix J: Summary of Respiratory-Related Changes in Older Adults

Decreases in:
- Vital capacity (VC: amount of air exhaled after a deep breath
- Inspiratory capacity (amount of air inhaled after exhaling)
- Elasticity of alveoli (ability of alveoli to open and close with ease)
- Oxygen in the arteries (PaO_2 levels)
- Ability to compensate under low oxygen levels (hypoxia)
- Cough reflex (related to possible changes in the medulla portion of the brain; medullar changes may influence the speed with which the older adult responds to hypoxia)
- Ciliary functioning (cilia are tiny hairs in the nasal passage and lung parenchyma, normally sifting small particles and bacteria from the lungs)

Increases in:
- Residual volume (air that pockets in the lungs)
- Stiffening of ribcage (related to excessive calcium in costral cartilidge between the ribs)

Appendix K: Summary of Cardiovascular Age-Related Changes in Older Adults

Decreases in:
- Release of calcium in the heart, prolonging contraction during systole
- Cardiac output at rest—*slight* decrease (mixed research results)
- Baroreceptor sensitivity (baroreceptor cells help regulate blood pressure), possibly readjusted as a result of a thicker, stiffer aorta and overall aging of nerve cells
- Left ventricular filling in diastole
- Hematocrit, hemoglobin, lymphocytes are slightly decreased

Increases in:
- Calcification and stiffening of the heart valves (aortic and mitral)
- Thickness in left ventricle wall, small increase
- Increase in atria (slight) with late diastolic filling to compensate for slowing of left ventricular filling; may result in S4 sound (atrial gallop)
- Fibrous tissue in the heart
- Amyloid tissue in the heart (debatable whether this is part of normal aging)
- Systolic and diastolic murmurs from ineffective valve closure
- Vessel rigidity in aorta
- Peripheral vascular resistance (mixed research findings; same versus increases)
- Blood pressure, slight increase
- Blood coagulation
- Fatty cells in the sinoatrial (SA) node, replacing pacer cells
- Electrocardiographic abnormalities
  - PR and QT intervals increase
  - Propensity for arrythmias

Appendix L: Summary of Age-Related Musculoskeletal Changes

Decreases in:
- Height (range of 2 to 4 inches from spinal column)
- **Trabecular** and **cortical bone,** especially in vertebrae, wrist, and hip
- Overall movement (slows)
- Strength (varies)
  - ↓Type II muscle fibers and isometric strength
  - ↓high-speed performance
- ↓reflexes
- ↓lean body mass
- ↓joint capsule (at elbows, knees, and wrists)

Increases in:
- cartilage: ears and nose broadens
- calcium loss from bones
- flexion of joints (**ankylosis:** stiffening of ligaments and joints)
- pelvis widens (but shoulders narrow)
- muscular wasting
- subcutaneous fat, especially at hips and abdomen
- bony prominences (more notable)
- resting tremors
- no change in long bones

Appendix M: Summary of Age-related Neurological Changes

- Brain decreases in size (by approximately 7 percent)
- Loss of neurons in the brain (up to 20 percent)
- Possible decrease in cerebral blood flow
- Little decline in intellect
- Increase in serotonin, decrease in norepinephrine (possibly contributes to depression)
- Slowing in deep tendon reflexes
- Slowing in peripheral nerve conduction
- Decreased speed of motor coordination
- Overall decrease in autonomic and sympathetic nervous system functions
- **Hypothalamus** function: decreased control of thermoregulation
- Some memory changes:
- Losses in short-term memory
- Clarity of long-term memory
- Some difficulty learning new information and retaining it; holds implications for client teaching about medications, procedures, prevention, etc.

Appendix N: Abnormal Inspection and Palpation, Breast and Node Findings in an Older Woman

- Reddened areas (breast, nipple, axillae)
- Striae unilaterally over breast or axilla
  — darker color in dark-skinned-persons

  — lighter color in light-skinned persons
- Unilateral vascularity
- Edema and thickening of tissue
  — orange rind appearance (*peau d'orange*)
- Asymmetrical nipple direction
- Change in shape of nipple, erosion of nipple
- Dimpling or retraction of breast
- Lesions/masses
- Palpable nodes > 1 centimeter in diameter

Appendix O: Classification of Aphasias

Aphasia	Pathophysiology	Expression	Characteristics
Broca's aphasia	Motor cortex lesion, Broca's area	Expressive Nonfluent	Speech slow and hesitant, the client has difficulty in selecting and organizing words. Naming, word and phrase repetition, and writing impaired. Subtle defects in comprehension.
Wernicke's aphasia	Left hemisphere lesion in Wernicke's area	Receptive Fluent	Auditory comprehension impaired, as is content of speech. Client unaware of deficits. Naming severely impaired.
Anomic aphasia	Left hemisphere lesion in Wernicke's area	Amnesic Fluent	Client unable to name objects or places. Comprehension and repetition of words and phrases intact.

Aphasia	Pathophysiology	Expression	Characteristics
Conduction aphasia	Lesion in the arcuate fasciculus, which connects and transports messages between Broca's and Wernicke's areas	Central Fluent	Client has difficulty repeating words, substitutes incorrect sounds for another (e.g., *dork* for *fork*).
Global aphasia	Lesions in the frontal-temporal area	Mixed Fluent	Both oral and written comprehension severely impaired, naming, repetition of words and phrases, ability to write impaired.
Transcortical sensory aphasia	Lesion in the periphery of Broca's and Wernicke's areas (watershed zone)	Fluent	Impairment in comprehension, naming, and writing. Word and phrase repetition intact.
Transcortical motor aphasia	Lesion anterior, superior, or lateral to Broca's area	Nonfluent	Comprehension intact. Naming and ability to write impaired. Word and phrase repetition intact.

Appendix P: Suspected Physiological Factors Related to Mental Health Changes in the Older Adult

- Decrease in large neurons
- Decrease in brain volume and brain weight
- Some decrease in short-term memory; long-term memory stays about the same
- Increase in reaction time to external stimuli
- Mild changes in sense of spatial accuracy and spatial relationships

■ SUSPECTED PSYCHOSOCIAL AND SPIRITUAL FACTORS ASSOCIATED WITH MENTAL HEALTH IN THE OLDER ADULT

- Multiple losses (loss of youth, loss of spouse, home, family, job, income)
- Loneliness versus sense of connection to others
- Hopelessness versus hopefulness
- Fear of death versus sense of peace
- Low self-worth versus positive self-esteem
- Negative coping mechanisms; i.e., substance abuse
- Meaninglessness in life versus sense of purposefulness

Appendix Q: Components of Mental Assessment in the Older Adult

*Inspection and analysis are the two major skills used.

Observe for:
- Physical appearance, grooming, and dressing (*not* a parameter when personal needs are provided by others; i.e. in a nursing home setting)
- Cultural and educational background
- Posture
- Movement
- Body language
- Facial expression
- Level of alertness and attentiveness

Analyze:
- Sleeping and eating patterns
- Medication usage
- Psychiatric history
- Laboratory test results
- Results of standardized cognition, orientation, judgment, and reasoning and depression scales (*interpret cautiously; many of these screening tests have minimal clinical value for older adult populations)

Appendix R: Working with Behaviors Associated with Dementia

- Assess and understand wandering behavior:
  - When does the person wander?
  - Where does the person wander?
  - Is there a pattern to the wandering?
  - Is the wandering meaningful? Aimless? Frantic?
  - Is the individual looking for something? Hiding/running from something?
  - Are others present when wandering occurs?
  - What is the degree of environmental stimuli when the person is wandering?
- *Do not use physical restraints* if at all possible because they increase agitation and fear, are dehumanizing, and *do not promote safety*. They contribute to immobility, constipation, pressure ulcers, and decline in cognition.
- Aim "control" at the environment not at the individual. Create an environment, that is 'wanderer-friendly,' with lounges, places to rest and socialize, nontoxic plants, appropriate lighting, and personally meaningful items. Hospitals and homes present difficult challenges in this area:
  - Specialized medical and surgical hospital units for older adults with dementia is an ideal solution to working *with* instead of *against* the acute needs of this group.
  - Home care nurses working with family members recommend home safety strategies so that the older adult can safely wander throughout his or her own home, night or day.
  - Specially trained volunteers and appropriate adult care centers throughout the community provide companionship, activities, and

care, again fitting the environment and stimuli to the person, not fitting the person to the environment.

- Try not to take aggressive behavior and angry statements personally. This is very difficult for nurses and others who have established long-standing relationships with an older adult with dementia. Seek out support groups and collegial support.
- Remain calm. Use a team approach that is nonviolent to help diffuse aggressive behaviors. Use pharmacological solutions as a last resort.
- Use gentle touch; do not rush the individual. Allow time for the older adult with dementia to acclimate to a new environment.
- Provide consistent caregivers when at all possible.
- Listen beyond what the person's words are saying; "listen" to feelings.
- Assure privacy, especially for those who exhibit socially inappropriate behaviors.
- Reflect on whether reality orientation is meaningful; validation therapy may be more suitable

Appendix S: NANDA Nursing Diagnoses 2005–2006

Activity Intolerance

Risk for Activity Intolerance

Impaired Adjustment

Ineffective Airway Clearance

Latex Allergy Response

Risk for Latex Allergy Response

Anxiety

Death Anxiety

Risk for Aspiration

Risk for Impaired Parent/Infant/Child Attachment

Autonomic Dysreflexia

Risk for Autonomic Dysreflexia

Disturbed Body Image

Risk for Imbalanced Body Temperature

Bowel Incontinence

Effective Breastfeeding

Ineffective Breastfeeding

Interrupted Breastfeeding

Ineffective Breathing Pattern

Decreased Cardiac Output

Caregiver Role Strain

Risk for Caregiver Role Strain

Impaired Verbal Communication

Readiness for Enhanced Communication

Decisional Conflict (Specify)

Parental Role Conflict

Acute Confusion

Chronic Confusion

Constipation

Perceived Constipation

Risk for Constipation

Defensive Coping

Ineffective Coping

Readiness for Enhanced Coping

Ineffective Community Coping

Readiness for Enhanced Community Coping

Compromised Family Coping

Disabled Family Coping

Readiness for Enhanced Family Coping

Risk for Sudden Infant Death Syndrome

Ineffective Denial

Impaired Dentition

Risk for Delayed Development

Diarrhea

Risk for Disuse Syndrome

Deficient Diversional Activity

Energy Field Disturbance

Impaired Environmental
  Interpretation Syndrome

Adult Failure to Thrive

Risk for Falls

Dysfunctional Family Processes:
  Alcoholism

Interrupted Family Processes

Readiness for Enhanced Family
  Processes

Fatigue

Fear

Readiness for Enhanced Fluid Balance

Deficient Fluid Volume

Excess Fluid Volume

Risk for Deficient Fluid Volume

Risk for Imbalanced Fluid Volume

Impaired Gas Exchange

Anticipatory Grieving

Dysfunctional Grieving

Risk for Dysfunctional Grieving

Delayed Growth and Development

Risk for Disproportionate Growth

Ineffective Health Maintenance

Health-Seeking Behaviors (Specify)

Impaired Home Maintenance

Hopelessness

Hyperthermia

Hypothermia

Disturbed Personal Identity

Functional Urinary Incontinence

Reflex Urinary Incontinence

Stress Urinary Incontinence

Total Urinary Incontinence

Urge Urinary Incontinence

Risk for Urge Urinary Incontinence

Disorganized Infant Behavior

Risk for Disorganized Infant Behavior

Readiness for Enhanced Organized
  Infant Behavior

Ineffective Infant Feeding Pattern

Risk for Infection

Risk for Injury

Risk for Perioperative-Positioning
  Injury

Decreased Intracranial Adaptive
  Capacity

Deficient Knowledge

Readiness for Enhanced Knowledge
  (Specify)

Risk for Loneliness

Impaired Memory

Impaired Bed Mobility

Impaired Physical Mobility

Impaired Wheelchair Mobility

Nausea

Unilateral Neglect

Noncompliance

Imbalanced Nutrition: Less than Body
  Requirements

Imbalanced Nutrition: More than
  Body Requirements

Readiness for Enhanced Nutrition

Risk for Imbalanced Nutrition: More
  than Body

Requirements

Impaired Oral Mucous Membrane

Acute Pain

Chronic Pain

Readiness for Enhanced Parenting

Impaired Parenting

Risk for Impaired Parenting

Risk for Peripheral Neurovascular Dysfunction

Risk for Poisoning

Post-Trauma Syndrome

Risk for Post-Trauma Syndrome

Powerlessness

Risk for Powerlessness

Ineffective Protection

Rape-Trauma Syndrome

Rape-Trauma Syndrome: Compound Reaction

Rape-Trauma Syndrome: Silent Reaction

Impaired Religiosity

Readiness for Enhanced Religiosity

Risk for Impaired Religiosity

Relocation Stress Syndrome

Risk for Relocation Stress Syndrome

Ineffective Role Performance

Sedentary Life Style

Bathing/Hygiene Self-Care Deficit

Dressing/Grooming Self-Care Deficit

Feeding Self-Care Deficit

Toileting Self-Care Deficit

Readiness for Enhanced Self-Concept

Chronic Low Self-Esteem

Situational Low Self-Esteem

Risk for Situational Low Self-Esteem

Self-Mutilation

Risk for Self-Mutilation

Disturbed Sensory Perception (Specify: Visual, Auditory, Kinesthetic, Gustatory, Tactile, Olfactory)

Sexual Dysfunction

Ineffective Sexuality Patterns

Impaired Skin Integrity

Risk for Impaired Skin Integrity

Sleep Deprivation

Disturbed Sleep Pattern

Readiness for Enhanced Sleep

Impaired Social Interaction

Social Isolation

Chronic Sorrow

Spiritual Distress

Risk for Spiritual Distress

Readiness for Enhanced Spiritual Well-Being

Risk for Suffocation

Risk for Suicide

Delayed Surgical Recovery

Impaired Swallowing

Effective Therapeutic Regimen Management

Ineffective Therapeutic Regimen Management

Readiness for Enhanced Management of Therapeutic Regimen

Ineffective Community Therapeutic Regimen Management

Ineffective Family Therapeutic Regimen Management

Ineffective Thermoregulation

Disturbed Thought Processes

Impaired Tissue Integrity

Ineffective Tissue Perfusion (Specify Type: Renal, Cerebral, Cardiopulmonary, Gastrointestinal, Peripheral)

Impaired Transfer Ability

Risk for Trauma

Impaired Urinary Elimination

Readiness for Enhanced Urinary Elimination

Urinary Retention

Impaired Spontaneous Ventilation

Dysfunctional Ventilatory Weaning
  Response

Risk for Other-Directed Violence

Risk for Self-Directed Violence

Impaired Walking

Wandering

Appendix T: Preparation for NCLEX

*A new graduate from an educational program that prepares registered nurses will take the NCLEX, the national nursing licensure examination prepared under the supervision of the National Council of State Boards of Nursing. NCLEX is taken after graduation and prior to practice as a registered nurse. The examination is given across the United States. Graduates submit their credentials to the state board of nursing in the state in which licensure is desired. Once the state board accepts the graduate's credentials, the graduate can schedule the examination. This examination ensures a basic level of safe registered nursing practice to the public. The examination follows a test plan formulated on four categories of client needs that registered nurses commonly encounter. The concepts of the nursing process, caring, communication, cultural awareness, documentation, self-care, and teaching/learning are integrated throughout the four major categories of client needs (Table T-1).

■ TOTAL NUMBER OF QUESTIONS ON NCLEX

Graduates may receive anywhere from 75 to 265 questions on the NCLEX examination during their testing session. Fifteen of the questions are questions that are being piloted to determine their validity for use in future NCLEX examinations. Students cannot determine whether they passed or failed the NCLEX examination from the number of questions they receive during their session. There is no time limit for each question, and the maximum time for the examination is 5 hours. A 10-minute break is mandatory after 2 hours of testing. An optional 10-minute break may be taken after another 90 minutes of testing.

Each test question has a test item and four possible answers. If the student answers the question correctly, a slightly more difficult item will follow, and the level of difficulty will increase with each item until the candidate misses an item. If the student misses an item, a slightly less difficult item will follow, and the level

*The future belongs to those who believe in the beauty of their dreams. (Eleanor Roosevelt)

TABLE T–1   NCLEX Test Plan: Client Needs

Client Needs Tested	Percent of Test Questions
Safe, effective care environment:	
Management of care	7–13%
Safety and infection control	5–11%
Physiologic integrity:	
Basic care and comfort	7–13%
Pharmacological and parenteral therapies	5–11%
Reduction of risk potential	12–18%
Physiological adaptation	12–18%
Psychosocial integrity:	
Coping and adaptation	5–11%
Psychosocial adaptation	5–11%
Health promotion and maintenance:	
Growth and development through the life span	7–13%
Prevention and early detection of disease	5–11%

of difficulty will decrease with each item until the student has answered an item correctly. This process continues until the student has achieved a definite passing or definite failing score. The least number of questions a student can take to complete the exam is 75. Fifteen of these questions will be pilot questions, and they will not count toward the student's score. The other 60 questions will determine the student's score on the NCLEX.

■ RISK FACTORS FOR NCLEX PERFORMANCE

Several factors have been identified as being associated with performance on the NCLEX examination. Some of these factors are identified in Table T-2.

■ REVIEW BOOKS AND COURSES

In preparing to take the NCLEX, the new graduate may find it useful to review several of the many NCLEX review books on the market. These review books often include a review of nursing content, or sample test questions, or both. They frequently include computer software disks with test questions for review. The test questions may be arranged in the review book by clinical content area, or they may be presented in one or more comprehensive

TABLE T–2   Factors Associated with NCLEX Performance

- HESI Exit Exam
- Mosby Assesstest
- NLN Comprehensive Achievement test
- NLN achievement tests taken at end of each nursing course
- Verbal SAT score
- ACT score
- High school rank and GPA
- Undergraduate nursing program GPA
- GPA in science and nursing theory courses
- Competency in American English language
- Reasonable family responsibilities or demands
- Absence of emotional distress
- Critical thinking competency

examinations covering all areas of the NCLEX. Listings of these review books are available at *www.amazon.com.* It is helpful to use several of these books and computer software when reviewing for the NCLEX.

NCLEX review courses are also available. Brochures advertising these programs are often sent to schools and are available in many sites nationwide. The quality of these programs can vary, and students may want to ask former nursing graduates and faculty for recommendations.

■ THE NLN EXAMINATION AND THE HESI EXIT EXAM

Many nursing programs administer an examination to students at the completion of their nursing program. Two of these exams are the NLN Achievement test and the HESI Exit Exam. New graduates will want to review their performance on any of these exams because these results will help identify their weaknesses and help focus their review sessions.

Students who examine their feedback from the NLN examination or the HESI Exit Exam have important information that can help them focus their review for the NCLEX. A strategy for examining this feedback and organizing this review is outlined in the following section.

■ ORGANIZING YOUR REVIEW

In preparing for NCLEX, identify your strengths and weaknesses. If you have taken the NLN examination or the HESI Exit Exam, note any content strength and weakness areas. Additionally, note any nursing program course or clinical content areas in which you scored below a grade of B. Purchase one or more of the NCLEX review books. It is useful to review questions developed by different authors. Review content in the review books in any of your weak content areas.Take a comprehensive exam in the review book or on the computer software disk and analyze your performance. Try to answer as many questions

TABLE T–3   Preparation for the NCLEX Test

Name: _____

Strengths: _____

Weak content areas identified on NLN examination or HESI Exit Exam:
_____
_____
_____

Weak content areas identified by yourself or others during formal nursing education program (include content areas in which you scored below a grade of B in class or any factors from Table T-2):
_____
_____
_____

Weak content areas identified in any area of the NCLEX test plan, including the following:
   Safe, effective care environment

   Physiological integrity

   Psychosocial integrity

   Health promotion and maintenance

Weak content areas identified in any of the top 10 patient diagnoses in each of the following:
   Adult health

   Women's health

   Mental health nursing

   Children's health
   (Consider the 10 top medications, diagnostic tools and tests, treatments and procedures used for each of the ten diagnoses.)

Weak content areas identified in the following:
   Therapeutic communication tools

   Defense mechanisms

   Growth and development

   Other

correctly as you can. Be sure to actually practice taking the examinations. Do not just jump ahead to look at the section on correct answers and rationales before answering the questions if you want to improve your examination performance.

Next, once you have completed the comprehensive examination, review the answers and rationales for any weak content areas and take another comprehensive exam. Repeat this process until you are doing well in all clinical content areas and in all areas of the NCLEX examination plan.

Finally, do a general review of the top 10 patient diseases, medications, diagnostic tests, and nursing procedures in each major nursing content area, as well as defense mechanisms, communication tips, and growth and development. Practice visualization and relaxation techniques as needed. These strategies will assist you in conquering the three areas necessary for successful test taking—anxiety control, content review, and test question practice. Table T-3 will help organize your study.

■ WHEN TO STUDY

Identify your personal best time. Are you a day person? Are you a night person? Study when you are fresh. Arrange to study 1 or more hours daily. Use Table T-4 to organize your study if you have 1 month to go.

Students who use this technique should increase their confidence in their ability to do well on the NCLEX.

TABLE T–4   Organizing your NCLEX Study

Note your weaknesses identified in Table T-3.
Take a comprehensive exam from one of the review books and analyze your performance. Then, depending on this test performance and the weaknesses identified in Table T-3, your schedule could look like the following:
Day 1:   Practice adult health test questions. Score the test, analyze your performance, and review test question rationales and content weaknesses.
Day 2:   Practice women's health test questions. Repeat above process.
Day 3:   Practice children's health test questions. Repeat above process.
Day 4:   Practice mental health test questions. Repeat above process.
Day 5:   Continue with other weak content areas. Continue this process until you are doing well in all areas of the test.

Appendix U: Glossary

Abduction   movement away from the middle of the body.

Acrochordon   a benign outgrowth of skin commonly found on axillae, eyelids, and neck; skin tag.

Acromegaly   a condition of enlarged and elongated bones associated with hypersecretion of the human growth hormone.

Actinic keratoses   a skin lesion associated with overexposure to sunlight; premalignant.

Activities of Daily Living (ADLs) activities necessary for living, including bathing, dressing, feeding, grooming, transferring, and toileting.

Adduction   movement toward the middle of the body.

Adnexa   Fallopian tubes, ovaries, and adjacent ligaments.

Advance directives   specific directives made out while a person is competent and included in a legal document that outlines one's wishes in the event of debilitating illness.

Adventitious breath sounds   abnormal additional breath sounds (wheezes, crackles, rhonchi).

Affective   having to do with mood.

Ageusia   loss of ability to taste.

Agraphia   inability to write.

Air conduction   sound traveling to the inner ear via air; air conduction takes longer than bone conduction.

Alexia   inability to understand the meaning of a word/sentences.

Alveoli   small packets of the lungs extending off the bronchioles.

Alzheimer's disease (AD)   a chronic, progressive, irreversible form of dementia.

Andropause   male stage of life similar to menopause, occurring around 50 years of age, with reduction in male hormones (testosterone).

Anesthesia   loss of sensation.

Angle of Louis   manubriosternal juncture; where the manubrium and sternum meet.

Ankylosis   joint stiffness and immobility.

Anorexia   no appetite due to malaise, fever, medication, depression, or psychological disorders.

Aneurysm   localized abnormal weakening or dilatation of a blood vessel, usually an artery.

Anus   opening of the rectum.

Aorta   begins at the upper portion of the left ventricle and extends as the major arterial network through the thorax, renal, abdominal, iliac, femoral, and tibial arteries.

Aphasia: expressive, receptive, and global

aphasia impaired ability to communicate.

expressive impaired ability to communicate verbally.

receptive impaired ability to understand.

global impaired ability to speak or understand.

Apical pulse pulse located at left mid-clavicular line at the 5th intercostal space, auscultated with a stethoscope; pulse heard at apex of the heart.

Apnea a period of breathing cessation lasting longer than 10 seconds.

Apraxia inability to actually verbalize a word that is thought of in the mind.

Aqueous humor liquid that passes through the posterior and anterior eye chambers.

Arcus senilis a white deposit of fat around the outer surface of the iris that does not normally interfere with vision.

Areola the circle of darker pigmentation around the nipple of each breast.

Arrhythmia irregular heart rhythm.

Arterial ulcers ulcers caused by arterial insufficiency; small, round, and smooth, often found on the foot and accompanied by pain and absent pulses (dorsalis pedis, posterior tibial, femoral, or popliteal).

Aspiration the inhaling of a substance other than air.

Assessment the first step in collecting subjective and objective data in the nursing process on which subsequent steps are based.

Astereognosis inability to identify objects by touch.

Atrioventricular node (AV node) controls electrical impulse of the heart, from atria to ventricles; 40 to 60 beats/minute is normal.

Atrium/atria upper two chambers of the heart.

Atrophic vaginitis inflammation of the vagina followed by menopause.

Auscultation investigation of the body by listening to its sounds.

Autonomic nervous system controls involuntary bodily functions.

Bartholin's cyst a cyst caused by blockage of fluid from Bartholin's glands, between the labia minora and hymenal ring.

Bell's Palsy facial paralysis on one side, from CN VII dysfunction; cause unknown.

Benign prostatic hyperplasia (BPH) increase in the number of cells in the prostate, often causing dysuria.

Blepharitis inflamed eyelids.

Blepharospasm a spasm of the orbicularis oculi muscle of the eye.

Blood pressure measure of the pressure from blood flowing in the large arteries.

Body transcendence versus body preoccupation one of three psychological developmental tasks of old age described by Robert Peck: emphasis on cognitive and social skills to allow compensation for physical limitations that are part of everyday life with aging.

Bone conduction sound traveling through the inner ear via bone; air conduction takes longer than bone conduction.

Bone mineral density (BMD) x-rays for determining density of bones; aids in the diagnosis of osteoporosis.

Borborygmi loud bowel sounds.

Bradykinesia extreme slowness of movement.

Brachial pulse   pulse palpated at the brachial artery.

Breast self-examination (BSE)   systematic and regular inspection and palpation of breasts and surrounding tissues performed by an individual on self.

Bronchial tubes   smaller tubes branching out from the bronchi.

Bronchophony   sound heard when client says "99" or "1–2–3"; determines if lungs are filled with air, fluid, or solid.

Bronchovesicular sounds   lung sound of moderate pitch and intensity heard at scapula and first or second intercostal spaces, equal on inspiration and expiration.

Bruits   abnormal swishing sounds upon auscultating veins/vessels.

Cachexia   muscle wasting.

Calorie   a unit of heat measurement.

Candida vaginosa   yeast cells that in excess create a white drainage and itching in the vaginal area.

Canker sore   red sore found in mouth or on lips.

Capillary refill test   pinching and blanching the finger nail bed and assessing the seconds it takes color to return.

Cardiac cycle   excitation of the heart allowing for the contraction and blood flow through the body.

Carotid pulse   pulse felt at the carotid artery.

Carpal tunnel syndrome   numbness in hand, wrist, and arm due to overuse and trauma to the hand muscles.

Cataract   opacity (cloudiness) of the eye's lens.

Central axillary nodes   lymph nodes found in the axillae.

Central nervous system   brain and spinal cord.

Cerebral vascular accident (CVA, stroke)   the obstruction of the blood and oxygen supply to a segment of the brain caused by a thrombus, an embolus, or bleeding.

Cerumen   ear wax.

Cervical smear   obtaining a lab specimen of the outer tissue at the inferior aspect of the uterus.

Chancre   red, round ulcer with raised edges and an indurated center.

Chandler's sign   tenderness of the cervix on palpation.

Cheyne-Stokes breathing   cyclical periods of breathing paired with no breathing.

Chief complaint   the main problem for which a person seeks health care.

Chlamydia   a bacteria that grows intracellularly and causes various lung and genital infections.

Circumlocution   unable to answer a question/topic; "circling around" a topic.

Clicks and gurgles   sounds heard in the abdomen connoting peristalsis (movement of food and gastric juices through the digestive tract).

Clitoris   located at the superior aspect of the vulva between the labia minora; contains erectile tissue with numerous nerve endings.

Cognition   the mental capacity characterized by recognition, memory, processing, learning, and judgment.

Colostomy   surgical opening of the colon to the external abdomen.

Complete health history   detailed past and present health history of a client.

Confabulation   a "making up" of answers when memory fails.

Conjunctivitis   inflammation of the conjunctiva of the eye due to infection or trauma.

Cooper's ligaments   ligaments that provide support to breast tissue; extend vertically through the fascia to inner skin layer through the breast.

Coronary arteries   the two major arteries, left and right, which feed blood to the myocardium.

Cortical bone   outer layer of bone.

Costal angle   angle where the costal margins meet at the sternum.

Crackles   a snapping sound heard on lung auscultation in a person who has atelectasis or other situations of alveolar closure. Formerly called rales. A similar sound can be obtained by twisting and rubbing your hair right behind the ear.

Cranial nerves   the twelve pairs of nerves emanating from the brain.

Crepitus   a grating sound as in bone against bone.

Crohn's disease   chronic inflammation of the bowel.

Cullen's sign   bluish color around umbilicus suggesting peritoneal bleeding.

Cuticle (nail)   tissue between the nail bed and nail.

Cystocele   anterior vaginal wall protrusion.

Deep tendon reflexes (DTR)   reflexes deep within the tendons, tested to assess central nervous system function.

Deep vein thrombosis (DVT)   a clot or thrombus occurring in the veins, usually in a leg.

Degenerative joint disease (DJD) wearing away at the joints resulting in stiffness and decreased range of motion.

Dehydration   excessive loss of water from body tissues.

Delirium   a rapid-onset state of confusion, disorientation, delusions, and sometimes hallucinations that is usually reversible with prompt appropriate treatment.

Dementia   a slow-onset, irreversible state of cognitive defects that can be the result of a medical condition or disease (such as Alzheimer's), substance reaction (such as long-term alcoholism), or a combination of these factors.

Depression   various degrees of feeling sad, helpless, hopeless, and perhaps suicidal.

Dermis   the second layer of skin.

Developmental task   a growth responsibility that occurs at a particular time in life.

Diaphoresis   excessive perspiration.

Dorsalis pedis pulse   pulse palpated at the top of the foot between the first and second toes.

Dyesthesia   misinterpretation of a stimulus, such as feeling a sharp stimulus as tingling.

Dysarthria   lack of muscular control in mouth, face, neck, throat, or brain needed to speak.

Dyspareunia   difficult, painful intercourse.

Dysphagia   difficulty in swallowing.

Dysphasia   speech impairment due to brain dysfunction.

Dysphonia   inability to make sounds of a word due to disease of the larynx.

Dyspnea   labored or difficult breathing.

Dysuria   difficulty urinating

Ecchymosis   "black-and-blue" mark; red-purple discoloration/bruise.

Eccrine   sweat glands.

Ectropion   eversion of the eyelids.

Edema   swelling; fluid excess.

Edentulous   being without natural teeth.

Ego differentiation versus work and role preoccupation   one of three psychological developmental tasks of old age described by Robert Peck: the development of valued alternatives in addition to one's work-role, acting to reaffirm self-worth.

Ego integrity versus despair   the eighth stage of development described by Eric Erikson as self-acceptance (ego integrity) versus dissatisfaction with life (despair).

Ego transcendence versus ego preoccupation   one of three psychological developmental tasks of old age described by Robert Peck: development of the ability to devote energies to the welfare of future generations without preoccupation with one's own death.

Egophony   sound produced when client says "ee;" used to assess presence of air, fluid, or solid in the lungs.

Elastosis   breakdown of connective tissue protein, elastin.

Elder mistreatment   acts of commission (intentional infliction of harm) or acts of omission (harm occurring through neglect) taken by a care-giver.

Elite older adult   person 85 years or older.

Enterostomal therapy nurse (ETN)   a nurse that specializes in ostomy care.

Entropion   eyelids that turn in causing the possibility of infection in the eye.

Epidermis   outer layer of skin.

Episodic health history   a specific, problem-generated client history, usually narrow and pertinent to the issue at hand.

Erythema   redness of the skin.

Estrogen replacement therapy (ERT)   hormone therapy given after menopause when the natural production of estrogen decreases.

Evaluation   the final step of the nursing process that measures the client's degree of goal achievement.

Exophthalmos   excessive protrusion of the eye.

External rotation   turning outward.

Extrapyramidal   outside the tracts of the central nervous system; emanates from the cortical and subcortical motor area structures of the brain.

Failure to Thrive (FTT)   in the absence of physiological etiology, the syndrome of overall decline, weight loss, and hopelessness thought to be caused by psychological deprivation.

Fall Efficacy Scale (FES)   a self-appraisal instrument to assess fall risk.

Femoral pulse   the pulse palpated at the femoral artery.

Food Guide Pyramid   guideline to improve food choices based on low-fat, high-fiber intake.

Forward flexion   bending limb, body, or joint forward.

Fovea centralis   middle of the macula that allows for sharpness of sight.

Functional status   ability of a person to carry out ADLs, IADLs, and social activities.

Gastrocsophogeal reflex disorder (GERD)   persistent reflux of the stomach contents into the esophagus.

Genogram   a diagrammatic display of a person's family health history.

Genitalia   male and female reproductive organs.

Gerontology   an interdisciplinary study of the process of aging.

Gerontological nursing   the holistic nursing care of sick and well older adults.

Gingivitis   inflammation of the gums.

Glasgow Coma Scale   widely used scale for grading neurological response.

Glaucoma   an eye disease characterized by increased intraocular pressure; it can cause blindness without treatment.

Goiter   enlarged thyroid.

Gonorrhea   a sexually transmitted disease caused by the bacteria *Neissera gonorrhoeae.*

Graves' Disease disease of hyper-thyroidism, with weight loss, heat intolerance, and eye and dermal involvement.

Gynecomastia collection of adipose tissue at the site of male breast tissue.

Heaves lifting of the cardiac area due to increased workload on the heart.

Heberden's nodes node thickening and enlargement at the distal phalanges of the fingers.

Hemorrhoids swelling of the hemorrhoidal veins in the rectum resulting in difficulty having a bowel movement.

Hepatic pertaining to the liver.

Herpes simplex caused by the virus of same name and resulting in eruption of vesicles in the oral area.

Hiatal hernia protrusion of a portion of the stomach through the diaphragm.

Hirschberg test symmetrical reflection of light off the cornea.

Hirsutism excessive body hair growth.

Hierarchy of needs a hierarchical framework consisting of five levels developed by Abraham Maslow to explain a person's level of functioning.

Homan's sign quick dorsiflexion of the foot resulting in pain (suggests venous thrombosis in the calf) or no pain.

Hordeolum a sty located in the eyelid.

Hormone replacement therapy (HRT) the use of hormones such as estrogen, progesterone, and testosterone (in small amounts) to supplement and eventually replace the natural ones that decline with menopause. Estrogen HRT is believed to prevent osteoporosis and reduce the incidence of heart disease in postmenopausal women.

Hydrocele the collection of fluid, especially in a cavity (such as the tunica vaginalis of the testis).

Hyperesthesia excessive sensitivity to touch.

Hyperextension extreme extension.

Hyperthyroidism the thyroid's over-secretion of thyroxine.

Hypoesthesia reduced sense of touch.

Hypogeusia reduction in the ability to taste.

Hypothalamus controls metabolic functions, fluid balance, body temperature, and hormonal balance.

Hypothyroidism reduced thyroid secretion requiring hormone replacement therapy.

Iatrogenic complication or disease caused by medical treatment and/or health care providers.

Ileostomy surgical opening and fecal drainage from the abdominal wall at the ileum.

Implementation portion of the nursing process focused on nursing interventions or approaches to facilitate the client's goal accomplishment.

Infraclavicular nodes lymph nodes located at the cavities of the clavicles.

Inorgasmia inability to experience an orgasm.

Isolated systolic hypertension a specific type of high blood pressure.

Inspection the skill of detailed and specific observation to assess an individual's health.

Instrumental Activities of Daily Living (IADL) managing money, shopping, housekeeping, preparing meals, and taking medications correctly.

Interdisciplinary approach/care care of geriatric patients requiring complex systems that involve numerous services and therapies. It is usually made up of health care providers (physicians, nurses, social workers, dietitians, psychologists, and others in the health care field).

Internal rotation turning inward.

Intervention   a purposeful nursing action focused at a positive client outcome.

IOP (intraocular pressure)   pressure within the eye, not related to blood pressure.

Iris   "eye color" of the eye; front portion of the uveal tract of the eye.

Irritable bowel disease   pain and cramping in the small and large intestines; constipation alternating with diarrhea; triggered by anxiety and dietary habits.

Jugular vein pressure (JVP)   pressure in the jugular vein observed and measured with the client in a sitting position; a good indicator of central venous pressure.

Kegel exercises   contracting exercises of the perineum to help treat urinary incontinence.

Korotkoff sounds   alteration in sounds as blood pressure cuff inflates around the arm.

Kussmaul's breathing   increase in rate and depth of respiration, as in diabetic ketoacidosis.

Kyphosis   "humpback"; convexation of the spine.

Lacrimal gland   gland in the eye that secretes tears.

Lateral nodes   lymph nodes located alongside body landmarks.

Left ventricular hypertrophy (LVH)   enlargement of the left ventricle of the heart.

Leukoplakia   white patches on tongue or cheeks.

Level of consciousness (LOC)   degree to which an individual manifests alertness; ranges from alert to comatose.

Life review   systematically evaluating one's successes and failures in life, with professional help, to resolve conflicts and prepare for death. Butler's concept that states that it is the awareness of one's own death that elicits an evaluation of one's life and how one has lived it.

Lipoma   fatty tumor.

Lithotomy position   supine with knees bent.

Low-density lipids (LDL)   cholesterol that contributes to blockage of arteries and cardiovascular disease.

Lungs   the two spongy organs in the thoracic cavity used for breathing.

Lymph   nodes alkaline fluid-filled nodal network throughout the body cavities used to cleanse tissues and fight infection.

Malnutrition   inadequate amount and quality of food intake.

Manubrium   top of sternum.

Mastectomy   removal of breast or breast tissue.

McBurney's point   a point in the right lower quadrant of the abdomen situated in the area of the appendix.

Menopause   cessation of menses in women in their late 40s to mid-50s due mainly to decreased estrogen production.

Mental health   feelings of personal wellness and successful adaptation to the outside world.

Miotic   pupillary contraction.

Mitral valve   valve between left atrium and left ventricle.

Mononucleosis   caused by Epstein-Barr or other virus with increase in mononuclear leukocytes characterized by flu symptoms.

Murmur   abnormal blowing, hissing, or swishing sounds of the heart.

Mutual goal-setting   establishing a client's health care goals involving both client and health care team.

Mydriatic   causing pupillary dilation.

Myopia   able to see only a short distance due to faulty lens refraction.

Myxedema   swelling, specific to thyroid dysfunction.

Nail root   proximal part of the nail.

Nailbed   nail portion of the finger or toe.

Normal aging   aging-related changes that occur in the absence of disease.

Nursing diagnosis   the client problem, as identified using specific taxonomy.

Nutrition Screening Initiative (NSI)   government, American Dietetic Association, and American Academy of Family Physicians' joint effort in the early 1990s to promote better nutrition in the older adult population.

Nystagmus   involuntary movements of the eye.

Occipital area   back of head.

Occupational therapist   professional trained in facilitating self-care, work skills, and leisure activities to enhance client independence.

Olecranon process   bony parts of the elbow.

Ophthalmologist   physician specializing in eye diseases.

Ophthalmoscope   instrument used to inspect and examine the eye.

Optometrist   professional who treats visual abnormalities as determined per state regulation. Scope of practice is not as expansive as that of the ophthalmologist.

Orientation   awareness of person, place, and time in reality.

Orthopnea   a respiratory symptom in which the person breathes most comfortably when in an upright position.

Orthostatic hypotension   *see postural hypotension.*

Osteoarthritis   degeneration of joints related to wear and tear.

Osteomyelitis   bone infection.

Osteoporosis   weakening and hollowing (decrease in bone mass) of the bones.

Otoscope   instrument used to examine the ear.

Outcome   consequence of interventions.

Paget's disease   inflammation of bones and a thickening and softening of bones; sometimes a bowing of legs.

Pain assessment   assessment that includes measures of pain intensity and pain experience, a combination that is important in evaluating chronic pain.

Pain, chronic   pain that extends past the normally expected time of healing. Pain that extends 3 months is commonly accepted as chronic within a clinical context, whereas 6 months is preferred for research purposes.

Palpation   understanding the body through deep and light touch.

Papanicolaou test   a diagnostic test of the cervix to determine abnormal conditions such as cancer.

Papilloma   superficial tumor.

Paranoid   suspicious thoughts and delusions characterized by intense feelings of persecution and threatening hallucinations.

Parasympathetic nervous system   includes cranial and sacral nerves.

Paresthesia   numbness or tingling; an abnormal sensation.

Parietal area   part of brain controlling somatic and sensory feelings.

Parkinson's disease   a neurological deficiency of dopamine, which results in a variety of symptoms, primarily tremor, muscle rigidity, and slow movement.

Paroxysmal nocturnal dyspnea (PND)   severe respiratory distress at night while sleeping flat, relieved by sitting up, and due to left side heart failure.

Pathological aging   age-related changes that are primarily a function of underlying disease states and are therefore not normal.

Pathological reflexes abnormal reflexes.

Pectoral nodes lymph nodes surrounding the pectoral area.

Peptic ulcer disease stomach, duodenal, or jejunal ulcer.

Percussion tapping parts of the body to determine abnormal versus normal conditions by sounds.

Pericardial friction rub sound heard during inspiration caused by an inflamed pericardium.

Perineum external area between vulva and anus, or scrotum and anus.

Periodontal disease disease of the gums and alveolar bones of the mouth. The common cause of tooth loss in older people. Can be prevented with proper care.

Peripheral nervous system cranial and spinal nerves.

Peritoneum lining of the abdominal cavity.

Periungual tissue tissue around the nail.

Pharmacokinetics the absorption, distribution, metabolism, and excretion of drugs in the body.

Physical therapist professional who focuses on rehabilitation and restoration of function emphasizing muscles and bones.

Planning aspect of nursing process that focuses on planning for actual care.

Plantar reflex foot reflex.

Pleural friction rub inflammation of the pleura resulting in a grating sound upon auscultation.

Polypharmacy the administration of multiple prescription and nonprescription medications simultaneously; often seen with older persons resulting in increased adverse effects.

Popliteal pulse pulse located behind knees.

Posterior tibial pulse pulse located at back of foot adjacent to Achilles tendon.

Postural hypotension a condition in which the blood pressure falls when changing to an upright position, resulting in dizziness or fainting.

Precordium term connoting frontal area over heart and thorax.

Presbycusis decreased ability to hear as one ages.

Presbyopia increased farsightedness (impaired near vision) in later middle age.

Pressure ulcer sore created mainly by pressure constricting blood flow to an area.

Pronator drift unilateral drift in one arm when client closes eyes and holds arms out, due to neurological problem such as stroke.

Prostate specific antigen (PSA) a screening blood test that indicates an abnormal condition of the prostate, especially cancer.

Pruritis excessive itching.

Psychotropics mood-altering drugs.

Pterygium yellow thickening of the conjunctiva.

Ptosis drooping eyelid.

Pulmonic area auscultated at second intercostal space left of the sternum.

Pulsation rhythmic beating or throbbing.

Pulse rhythmic movement of blood flow through arteries.

Pulse deficit when radial pulse is less than apical pulse.

Pulse oximetry indirect measurement of oxygenation via a sensor on the outside of the body: often on ear lobe or finger.

Quality of life　what the individual determines is quality relative to her or his life.

Radial pulse　pulse located at the wrist at the base of the thumb.

Rales　*see* crackles.

Range of motion (ROM)　the range of movement of a joint; the "north-south-east-west" movement of limbs; may be active (self-movement) or passive (movement of a limb by another).

Rate　the numerical counting or speed of something such as heart beats per minute.

Reminiscence therapy　thinking and talking about mostly pleasant memories from the past.

Respiration　inhale-exhale breathing cycle.

Rectocele　protrusion through the vagina of the posterior vaginal wall.

Red reflex　shining light from the ophthalmoscope into the pupil onto the retina, which should reflect a light reflection.

Registered Dietician (R.D.)　the health professional whose expertise is in nutrition.

Required Dietary Allowances (RDA)　national recommendations for the daily intake of certain vitamins and minerals by age groups.

Review of systems (ROS)　client's subjective response to body system questions, which must be confirmed through examination and other data.

Rhythm　regularity in sound or movement, such as in a beating heart or breathing.

Ringworm　skin infection caused by various fungi, noted by a red-ringed patch of vesicles that itch.

Rinne test　use of a tuning fork to test for bone versus air conduction through the ear canal.

Scapula　flat, triangular bone at the posterior shoulders.

Scoliosis　curvature of the spine, laterally.Sebaceous glands glands that secrete sebum, a fatty oil.

Sebaceous glands　glands that secrete sebum, a fatty oil.

Seborrhea　dandruff.

Seborrheic keratosis　benign skin tumor.

Sebum　the body's natural oil.

Self-care　ability to meet one's own daily needs.

Self-care deficit　various degrees of inability to care for self.

Self-esteem　individual's sense of self-worth.

Self-neglect　inability to provide self-care to meet basic needs.

Senescence　the process of aging; the biological, physiological, sociological, and psychological changes that accompany the aging process.

Sensory impairment　decrease in one or more of the five senses (sight, hearing, taste, smell, touch).

Sexually transmitted diseases (STDs)　diseases transmitted through oral/genital contact.

Sinoatrial node (SA node)　nerves in the heart that initiate electrical activity needed for cardiac muscle contraction.

Sleep apnea　cessation of respiration during sleep lasting longer than 10 seconds.

Snellen chart　chart used to test vision; ranges from small to large letters. Social roles the activities, rights, and responsibilities that accompany a particular position in society. Social skills interactional techniques required for integration into society. Social support a person, agency, or organization from which one receives individual assistance, encouragement, and comfort when needed.

Speculum   instrument used to view body cavity, such as bivalve speculum to view the vagina.

Speech/language pathologist   a professional who specializes in diagnosis and treatment of speech and language abnormalities.

Spermatocele   tumor located in the epididymis.

Spinal processes   bony protrusions from the vertebrae of the spine.

Spiritual well-being   the affirmation of life in a relationship with a God, self, community, and environment that nurtures and celebrates wholeness.

Spirituality   belief in a greater life form and existence.

Stereognosis   identification of objects by touch.

Sternocleidomastoid   muscle at the inner part of the clavicle. Sternum flat bone dividing the anterior thorax.

Subcutaneous tissue   tissue directly beneath the epidermis.

Subluxation   partial dislocation of a bone.

Subscapular nodes   lymph nodes located in the cavity below the shoulder blades.

Sundown syndrome   increased degree of confusion and disorientation that occurs in older persons with dementia in the late afternoon or early evening.

Sunrise syndrome   decreased cognitive functioning early in the morning.

Superficial reflexes   reflexes related to surface nerves.

Supraclavicular nodes   lymph nodes located above the clavicles.

Sympathetic nervous system   starts from thoracic and lumbar spine; when stimulated, increases heart rate, dilates pupils, and increases epinephrine and norepinephrine in response to stressors.

Tactile fremitus   vibrations felt when hands are placed on client's chest. Tail of Spence upper outer part of the chest, which extends into the axilla.

Tardive dyskinesia   abnormal movements of the tongue, neck, fingers, trunk, and legs caused by some antipsychotic medications.

Telangiectasia   lesion consisting of small blood vessels.

Temperature   body heat measured in Fahrenheit or Celsius units. Temporal area below frontal lobe of brain; controls some auditory functions.

Temporal pulse   pulse located at temple.

Temporomandibular joint (TMJ)   between mandible and temporal bones; if inflamed or stiff, creates pain and clicking in the jaw area. Testicular torsion a twisting or strangulation of the testes causing circulatory blockage; emergency surgery is required.

Thalamus   mediates sensory stimuli, pain, temperature, and aspects of touch.

Thomas test   knee to chest movement while supine; remaining leg should stay flat on the examination table. Thorax chest cavity.

Thrills   quivering felt from a cardiac murmur.

Tinetti Balance and Gait Evaluation   a seventeen-item scored instrument used to assess gait plus balance; the lower the score, the greater the likelihood of imbalance.

Tonometry   measures intraocular pressure to detect glaucoma.

Torticollis   neck deformity, with head tilted to one side.

Trabecular bone   woven, meshed tissue found inside the bones.

Trachea   tubular structure from larynx to bronchi.

Tragus   protrusion at the external anterior ear.

Transient ischemic attack (TIA)   a stroke, which comes and goes (is transient); symptoms of a stroke that usually last 20 minutes to 24 hours and can be a predictor of a major stroke.

Tricuspid valve   heart valve between the right atrium and right ventricle.

Turgor   tautness; tension of the skin often referred to as skin turgor.

Tympany   hollow sound, like that made by beating on a drum.

Unna boot   layered gauze dressing of lower extremities used in treatment of venous leg ulcers.

Urethral meatus   opening of the bladder as it exits the body.

Urinary tract infection (UTI)   bacterial infection of the bladder, ureter, and/or kidneys.

Uvula   soft structure hanging at the soft palate in the back of the throat.

Vaginal introitus   entrance into the vagina.

Venous hum   continuous hum heard in veins; may suggest anemia.

Venous ulcers   sores usually found on the lower legs caused by venous insufficiency stasis.

Ventricle   two lower chambers of the heart; left chamber pumps blood to the aorta and out to the body; right chamber pumps blood to the pulmonary artery and lungs.

Vertebra prominens   7th cervical vertebra.

Vertigo   dizziness; feeling of motion and unbalance of equilibrium.

Vesicular sounds   soft, smooth sounds heard in normal lungs.

Vital signs   temperature, pulse, respiration, blood pressure, and degree of comfort/pain.

Weber test   tests for nerve or conductive hearing loss.

Wheezes   abnormal, high-pitched whistling breath sounds.

Xanthelasma   nodule found on eyelids near inner canthus.

Xerophthalmia   a sequence of abnormalities of increasing severity in the conjunctiva and cornea of the eye caused by vitamin A deficiency. Rare in the United States but common in Southeast Asia and parts of Africa and South America.

Xerosis   excessively dry skin.

Xiphoid process   protrusion at lower part of sternum; calcifies as people age.

Code Legend

NP	**Phases of the Nursing Process**
As	Assessment
An	Analysis
Pl	Planning
Im	Implementation
Ev	Evaluation

CN	**Client Need**
Sa	Safe Effective Care Environment
Sa/1	Management of Care
Sa/2	Safety and Infection Control
He/3	Health Promotion and Maintenance
Ps/4	Psychosocial Integrity
Ph	Physiological Integrity
Ph/5	Basic Care and Comfort
Ph/6	Pharmacological and Parenteral Therapies
Ph/7	Reduction of Risk Potential
Ph/8	Physiological Adaptation

CL	**Cognitive Level**
K	Knowledge
Co	Comprehension
Ap	Application
An	Analysis

SA	**Subject Area**
1	Medical-Surgical
2	Psychiatric and Mental Health
3	Maternity and Women's Health
4	Pediatric
5	Pharmacologic
6	Gerontologic
7	Community Health
8	Legal and Ethical Issues

Practice Test 1

1. A 92-year-old client is visibly upset and tells the nurse, "I want to talk with the head nurse, no, get me the supervisor and the director of nursing and the owner of this nursing home. I am mad!" The best initial response for the nurse to make is

    1. "Why do you want to talk with them?"
    2. "Don't be angry!"
    3. "Settle down or I'll have to call your daughter."
    4. "You seem upset."

2. The nurse is applying a lower leg brace to a 77-year-old client with hemiplegia. Which aspect of the client's condition is a priority for the nurse to consider when planning for the client's safety? The client

    1. cannot move one leg.
    2. is unable to use one hand and arm to help apply the brace.
    3. has difficulty fully extending the ankle.
    4. has no sensation in the leg where the brace is being applied.

3. When caring for an 85-year-old client who has just had a bronchoscopy under local anesthesia, the appropriate nursing intervention is to

    1. administer oxygen to the client.
    2. position the client in a prone position.
    3. explain that the client cannot have food or drink for several hours.
    4. have an emergency tracheostomy set nearby.

4. The nurse is caring for an 82-year-old client who is newly diagnosed with type II diabetes mellitus. Which of the following is the most appropriate nursing goal? The client will

   1. maintain nearly normal blood glucose levels.
   2. plan menus to fit the dietary prescription.
   3. demonstrate the proper insulin injection technique.
   4. demonstrate the correct technique for checking blood glucose levels.

5. Based on an understanding of hypertension and smoking, which of the following is the priority rationale for the nurse to instruct an older adult client to quit smoking?

   1. Smoking causes the arteries to constrict and raises blood pressure
   2. The tar in cigarette smoke causes changes in the lungs and bronchi
   3. Smoking residues build up in the bladder and can cause cancer
   4. The lungs are damaged by smoke and may develop cancer

6. The nurse is caring for an 86-year-old man who has a fractured pelvis and femur after a motor vehicle accident. After three days in the hospital, the client asks the nurse to go out dancing. Based on an understanding of the situation, the nurse identifies the best explanation for this behavior as the fact that the client

   1. has sexual feelings for the nurse.
   2. wants to get to know the nurse better.
   3. is attracted to the nurse.
   4. wants to be assured that healing will occur and dancing will be possible.

7. An 88-year-old client admitted to a long-term care facility becomes confused about place and time. The nurse starts a reality orientation plan, but when the client's perceptions are corrected the client becomes belligerent. At this point, it is most appropriate for the nurse to

   1. request an order for a sedative.
   2. continue to confront the client with reality.
   3. move the client to a different place in the facility.
   4. verbally express empathy with the client's misperceptions.

8. A client who has dementia is pacing aimlessly in a nursing facility. The client states a need to "go home" and is looking for the door. Initially, the nurse should

   1. assign a staff member to pace with the client and make sure there is no opportunity to leave the facility.

2. distract the client with an invitation to an activity, use the restroom, or eat a snack.

3. allow the client to act out feelings to determine what the priority needs are.

4. be accessible to set limits on the client's behavior as needed.

9. An older adult client confined to a room has little outside stimulation except for that provided by the health care team. The client becomes more quiet and distant. The nurse changes the plan of care to include more sensory stimulation. The best outcome measure would be that the client

1. interprets input appropriately when stimulated by the health care team.

2. approves of church member visits once a week to read scriptures.

3. calls the nurse by name.

4. is awake and alert on health care team visits and initiates conversation.

10. A 68-year-old client in a primary care clinic reports the sudden development of urinary incontinence, urgency, and "dribbling" on the way to the bathroom. The nurse recognizes that this problem is most likely related to

1. being obese.

2. having had multiple pregnancies.

3. a urinary tract infection.

4. receiving estrogen therapy.

11. Which of the following is the priority for the nurse to perform when a 93-year-old client is admitted with edema and congestive heart failure, but renal failure, and liver dysfunction have been ruled out?

1. Place the client on diuretics

2. Obtain a nutrition evaluation including protein intake

3. Increase the client's bed rest

4. Monitor the client's intake

12. The nurse visits an older adult couple living independently. The wife has dementia and the husband has recently been hospitalized for the repair of a fractured hip. He states, "I just can't take care of her anymore and I am afraid she will die without me." Which of the following is the best response by the nurse?

1. "Why don't you hire full-time live-in help?"

2. "She doesn't know you any more. She'll be OK."

3. "Can you live with family?"

4. "There are living arrangements where you can get help and be together."

13. An older adult who has recently been widowed has moved to an assisted living care center. Which of the following is an appropriate goal for meeting this client's developmental needs? The client will

    1. begin to lose a sense of independence and become more dependent in one month.

    2. express a satisfaction with the current living arrangement within two months.

    3. correct the cause of social isolation and make new friends in one week.

    4. use family for support and assistance with emotional needs in two weeks.

14. An 85-year-old client who lives alone and takes multiple drugs for the control of hypertension is admitted to an acute care unit. The client's daughter reports that confusion, disorientation, slurred speech, and changes in levels of consciousness have developed in the last two days. The nurse reports these clinical manifestations as indicative of

    1. Alzheimer's disease.

    2. delirium.

    3. dementia.

    4. amnesia.

15. Which of the following is a priority for the nurse to assess in an older adult client who was admitted and has multiple medical problems including emphysema, arthritis, and congestive heart failure?

    1. What drugs is the client taking?

    2. When did the client last see the physician?

    3. How has the client's appetite been?

    4. Does the client drive a car?

16. A 74-year-old male who has smoked cigarettes for 65 years tells the nurse his left foot is "bruised" and cold. The left foot is reddish purple, has a faint pedal pulse, and is cool and painful. The priority nursing intervention is

    1. treat this client for a venous insufficiency.

    2. report this as arterial insufficiency and a medical emergency.

    3. encourage the client to exercise the foot.

    4. apply a heating pad to the foot.

17. An older adult client who is obese has venous insufficiency and edema in the legs. Which of the following interventions is appropriate?

1. Position the legs in a downward position
2. Position the legs at heart level with compression stockings
3. Place the feet in warm water
4. Apply ice packs to the lower legs

ANSWERS AND RATIONALES

1. **4.** Asking a "why" question places the client in a defensive position. Telling a client not to be angry tells the client how and what to feel. Telling a client to settle down or the client's daughter will be called is a threat. The most appropriate response to clients who are upset is to allow them to explain their feelings. Stating, "You seem upset" acknowledges the client's feelings, facilitating further assessment.
   NP = An
   CN = Ph/8
   CL = An
   SA = 6

2. **4.** When planning for a hemiplegic client's safety, the priority is that there is no sensation in the leg where the brace is being applied. The fact that the client cannot move the leg, has difficulty extending the ankle, and is unable to use one hand and arm to help apply the brace are important considerations, but are not the priority.
   NP = An
   CN = Sa/1
   CL = An
   SA = 6

3. **3.** Following a bronchoscopy, it is important that the client not have anything to drink or eat until the gag and swallowing reflexes return. Oxygen is generally not necessary. A prone position is contraindicated, because it may cause the client to experience respiratory difficulty. Semi-Fowler's position is correct for a client after a bronchoscopy, to facilitate drainage of oral secretions. A tracheostomy set is not necessary following a bronchoscopy.
   NP = Pl
   CN = Ph/7
   CL = Ap
   SA = 6

4. **1.** An appropriate goal for a client with type 2 diabetes mellitus is to maintain a nearly normal blood glucose level. Planning menus, demonstrating proper insulin injection techniques, and demonstrating the correct technique for checking blood glucose levels are all outcome criteria.

NP = Ev
CN = Ph/8
CL = Ap
SA = 6

5. 1. Based on an understanding of hypertension and the effects of smoking on blood pressure, it would be a priority for the nurse to explain that smoking constricts the arteries and causes the blood pressure to rise.
NP = Pl
CN = Sa/1
CL = An
SA = 6

6. 4. A client with a fractured pelvis who asks the nurse to go out dancing is most likely assuming that the pelvis will heal and dancing once again will be possible. The client's behavior most likely is not related to sexual feelings or attraction. The client's behavior indicates feelings of insecurity after the injury.
NP = An
CN = Ph/8
CL = An
SA = 6

7. 4. Dealing with a client's feelings and frustrations is the priority when a client is confused and becomes belligerent. Expressing empathy opens the issues to discussion. A sedative would interfere with the client's adjustment and can increase the client's confusion. Further reality orientation and confrontation would make the client more belligerent. Moving the client would increase the confusion.
NP = Im
CN = Ph/8
CL = Ap
SA = 6

8. 2. A client who has dementia and is pacing aimlessly may be looking for something, perhaps the bathroom or food. Distraction or redirection is preferable to allowing the client to expend energy and become more agitated. Keeping the client safe is the priority, but assigning one staff member to pace with the client may not be possible. Redirection and distraction would not exacerbate the situation and cause a catastrophic event.
NP = Im
CN = Ph/8
CL = Ap
SA = 6

9. 4. An outcome should be stated as "The client will ·····" and should be measurable. Stimulation by the health care team is neither an outcome nor directly measurable. That the client approves of a visit does not correlate with the goal of sensory stimulation. That the client knows the nurse's name indicates recognition of the nurse, but does not directly relate to the goal. Only the statements that the client is awake and alert on health care team visits and initiates conversations are measurable.
NP = Ev
CN = Ph/8
CL = An
SA = 6

10. 3. A client who is suddenly experiencing urinary urgency, incontinence, and dribbling is most likely experiencing a urinary tract infection. Although being obese and having multiple pregnancies may result in similar clinical manifestations, neither would be a contributing factor at age 68 years. Oral estrogen therapy may be used in the treatment of stress incontinence, which occurs from thinning of the uterus wall and changes in the urethra during and after menopause.
NP = An
CN = Ph/8
CL = An
SA = 6

11. 2. When a client with congestive heart failure has edema but kidney and liver failure have been ruled out, an adequate protein intake is crucial for keeping water in the intravascular space. An evaluation of protein intake as well as serum albumin would indicate whether the edema results from inadequate protein.
NP = Im
CN = Sa/1
CL = Ap
SA = 6

12. 4. An older adult couple having trouble living independently for whatever reason should be told that there are living arrangements where help may be provided while staying together. This maintains open communication with the couple.
NP = An
CN = Ph/8
CL = An
SA = 6

13. 2. Clients should be able to meet their own emotional needs through friends, self, staff, and family. They should be independent and as autonomous as possible.

NP = Ev
CN = Ph/8
CL = An
SA = 6

14. 2. That an older adult client has developed confusion, disorientation, slurred speech, and changes in the level of consciousness within a period of time as short as two days indicates delirium. Alzheimer's disease and other forms of dementia occur over long periods of time. There is no reason to anticipate a finding of amnesia.
NP = An
CN = Ph/8
CL = Ap
SA = 6

15. 1. The priority in assessing any client who presents with multiple health problems is asking the client what drugs are being taken. Asking when the physician was last seen, how the appetite has been, and if the client is driving are all appropriate questions, but not the priority.
NP = As
CN = Ph/8
CL = An
SA = 6

16. 2. Because the foot is reddish purple and cool with a weak pulse, the insufficiency is arterial. If the foot had been warm and swollen, there might be a venous insufficiency. The viability of the foot is at risk, and this is a medical emergency.
NP = Im
CN = Sa/1
CL = Ap
SA = 6

17. 2. Placing the legs and feet in a dependent position or applying external heat with a heating pad will increase the swelling and edema in a client who has a venous insufficiency. In addition, the heating pad may cause burns to the fragile edematous tissue. The ice packs may decrease circulation and damage tissue.
NP = Im
CN = Ph/8
CL = Ap
SA = 6

HEALTH ISSUES OF THE OLDER ADULT - COMPREHENSIVE EXAM

1. When planning the care of a 98-year-old client with congestive heart failure, which of the following should the nurse perform to determine if the heart failure is right- or left-sided?

   1. Auscultate the lungs in all fields

   2. Listen to the mitral valve

   3. Feel for the point of maximal impulse on the client's chest

   4. Calculate the pulse pressure

2. Based on an understanding that the clinical manifestations of a medical condition may be different in an older person than in a younger person, the nurse evaluates an older adult to be experiencing a heart problem or pneumonia when which of the following are present?

   1. Incontinence

   2. Headache

   3. Restlessness and confusion

   4. Nausea and vomiting

3. Which of the following should the nurse assess first in a client with profound skeletal changes from osteoporosis? The ability to

   1. walk across the room.

   2. climb stairs.

   3. daily exercise.

   4. perform activities of daily living.

4. The nurse evaluates which of the following to be the priority issue for an older adult client who has a chronic or disabling joint or bone condition?
    1. Depression
    2. Pain
    3. Decreased financial security
    4. Loss of activity

5. The nurse is screening four clients for osteoporosis. Which of the following clients does the nurse determine to be at greatest risk for osteoporosis?
    1. An African-American woman
    2. A thin woman of north European descent
    3. An overweight Asian-American man
    4. A Native American woman

6. Which of the following should the nurse include in the environmental fall-risk assessment in an older client?
    1. Muscle strength
    2. Balance
    3. Gait
    4. Clutter and pets

7. The nurse evaluates which of the following to compromise the assessment of the respiratory function in an older adult?
    1. Increased anterior-posterior diameter of the chest
    2. Dehydration
    3. Hypertension
    4. Enlargement of the heart

8. The nurse should administer oxygen to a client with a chronic obstructive lung disease such as emphysema at what oxygen flow rate?
    1. 3 L/minute
    2. 6 L/minute
    3. 8 L/minute
    4. 12 L/minute

9. The registered nurse is making clinical assignments in a nursing facility. Which of the following assignments would be appropriate to delegate to team members?
    1. Unlicensed assistive personnel perform the activities of daily living for older adult clients

2. A licensed practical nurse develops a plan of care for an older adult client with congestive heart failure

3. Unlicensed assistive personnel perform active range-of-motion exercises on older adult clients

4. A licensed practical nurse evaluates an older adult client for readiness for discharge

ANSWERS AND RATIONALES

1. 1. To determine if the congestive heart failure is the result of a left- or right-sided failure, it is necessary to auscultate the lungs in all lung fields. Left-sided heart failure is manifested by fluid in the lungs resulting from blood backing up from the left ventricle.
    NP = Pl
    CN = Ph/8
    CL = Ap
    SA = 6

2. 3. Suddenly becoming incontinent may indicate a bladder infection in an older adult. A headache and vomiting are vague manifestations of many conditions. Restlessness and confusion are often indicators of hypoxia in the older adult.
    NP = Ev
    CN = Ph/8
    CL = An
    SA = 6

3. 4. In an advanced stage, osteoporosis affects the vertebral column. Although assessing the client's ability to walk, climb stairs, or perform daily exercise is important, the first assessment should be to evaluate the client's ability to perform activities of daily living. Maintaining the ability to perform activities of daily living will keep the client as independent as possible.
    NP = As
    CN = Sa/1
    CL = An
    SA = 6

4. 1. The client with a chronic or disabling joint or bone condition may experience chronic pain, decreased financial security, and a loss of activity. These all lead to depression, which is the priority. The depression directly affects the client's compliance with treatment.
    NP = Ev
    CN = Sa/1
    CL = An
    SA = 6

5. **2.** The thin, fair-skinned woman is at greatest risk for osteoporosis because of their fair skin and light weight. The darker the individual and the more muscle or even fat the individual carries, the stronger the bones.
NP = An
CN = Ph/8
CL = Ap
SA = 1

6. **4.** Even though muscle strength, balance, and gait are part of a fall-risk assessment, environmental risk factors, including clutter, throw rugs, electrical cords, and pets running loose, are important causes of falls in the home.
NP = As
CN = Ph/8
CL = An
SA = 6

7. **1.** In older adults, the bony structure of the chest may have changed over time as a result of retained air from chronic obstruction conditions. The round, barrel-shaped chest will make it harder to hear lung and heart sounds.
NP = Ev
CN = Ph/8
CL = Ap
SA = 6

8. **1.** In obstructive lung diseases, a higher-than-normal carbon dioxide level affects the client's respiratory drive. If that level is decreased rapidly by increasing the oxygen, the client may stop breathing. The safest range is 2 L to 3 L/minute. If the client requires more than that, intubation and mechanical ventilation may be necessary.
NP = Im
CN = Ph/8
CL = An
SA = 6

9. **1.** Unlicensed assistive personnel may perform the activities of daily living for older adult clients. Developing a plan of care and evaluating a client's readiness for discharge are tasks that should be performed by a registered nurse. Unlicensed assistive personnel should not perform active range-of-motion exercises on clients. This is a skill that should be performed by either a licensed practical nurse or a registered nurse.
NP = Pl
CN = Sa/1
CL = An
SA = 8

DELIRIUM AND DEMENTIA - COMPREHENSIVE EXAM

1. A physician caring for an 83-year-old client recommends to the family that a psychiatric consultation be performed to evaluate the client for depression. The family member asks the nurse, "Why is a psychiatric evaluation necessary? All old people are depressed because they are going to die soon." The priority response for the nurse to make initially is

   1. "Depression is not a normal part of aging."
   2. "Has your parent had many losses?"
   3. "Don't you see how depressed the client is?"
   4. "Has the client always been like this?"

2. An older adult is treated in the emergency department for burns sustained in a home fire. Abuse is ruled out. The client tells the nurse, "I must have left the stove on and my dinner in the skillet caught on fire. Then I couldn't find the number for the fire department. I just didn't know what to do." In addition to assessment of physical parameters, it is a priority that the nurse assess for

   1. the social support system.
   2. who else lives in the home.
   3. depression and cognitive function.
   4. community services available to assist the client in the home.

3. An older adult is found wandering on the street and is taken to a nearby emergency department. The client tells the nurse, "I know what you want. You're after my money. I'm the king and you must do what I say." Based on an understanding of delusions in the older adult, the nurse should assess for which of the following etiologies?

   1. Hypothermia
   2. Hypertension
   3. Dehydration
   4. Infection

4. The nurse should monitor an older adult who is receiving rivastigmine (Exelon) for which of the following adverse reactions?
   Select all that apply:
   [ ] 1. Hypotension
   [ ] 2. Anorexia
   [ ] 3. Weight gain
   [ ] 4. Abdominal pain
   [ ] 5. Urinary retention
   [ ] 6. Dizziness

5. An 85-year-old woman with dementia who is a nursing home resident asks the nurse repeatedly, "When will my husband be here to visit me today?" Her husband died 10 years ago. The appropriate response by the nurse is

   1. "I'm sorry but your husband died 10 years ago."
   2. "I don't think he will be able to visit today."
   3. "I understand you would like your husband here with you. How did you meet him?"
   4. "We'll have to wait and see if he can come today."

6. An older adult is experiencing an idiosyncratic reaction to an opioid prescribed for pain. The client is unsteady and laughing as if inebriated in this state of delirium. Providing a safe environment for the client is essential. A family member asks the nurse, "Will this go away? Or will he always be like this?" The priority response for the nurse to make is

   1. "This may be permanent and progress like dementia."
   2. "Delirium can be reversed if the cause is found and treated."
   3. "Drinking more water will make it go away sooner."
   4. "I will stay with him to keep him safe."

7. An older adult living in a nursing home who has been cognitively intact becomes very restless and agitated. Oxygen saturation is 80%, which is a change from 96% a day ago. Because of the sudden onset of the change in mental status and cognitive function, the nurse should

   1. administer oxygen at 2 L to 3 L/minute by nasal prongs.
   2. start an intravenous infusion of 5% dextrose in water.
   3. give the client orange juice orally.
   4. call an ambulance.

8. A previously cognitively intact older adult with type 1 diabetes mellitus becomes confused about person, place, and time. The client is irritable and insists on wearing a heavy coat indoors. Which of the following should the nurse perform first?

   1. Check the client's blood pressure
   2. Check the client's blood sugar
   3. Check the client's oxygen saturation
   4. Call the health care provider

ANSWERS AND RATIONALES

1. **1.** A commonly held myth is that depression is a normal part of aging and that older adults have many reasons to be depressed. By stating that

depression is not normal, the nurse is opening communication to further discussion.

NP = An
CN = Sa/1
CL = An
SA = 6

2. 3. Forgetfulness may be a manifestation of depression or dementia. The client's cognitive function and depression should be assessed. Some short-term memory loss, such as forgetting where the car keys are, is normal with aging.

NP = As
CN = Sa/1
CL = An
SA = 6

3. 3. An older adult client found wandering, who states, "You are only after my money and I am the king," is experiencing delusions. These delusions may be related to dehydration and a resulting hypernatremia.

NP = As
CN = Ph/8
CL = An
SA = 6

4. 2, 4, 6. Rivastigmine (Exelon) is used in the treatment of mild to moderate Alzheimer's disease. Adverse reactions to Exelon include anorexia, nausea, vomiting, abdominal pain, hypertension, weight loss, and dizziness.

NP = As
CN = Ph/6
CL = Ap
SA = 5

5. 3. The nurse should treat a client who has dementia and is asking when her dead husband is going to visit with compassion. Telling the resident that her husband died 10 years ago may cause her to argue and may precipitate a catastrophic reaction. She may grieve again and again every time she is told he is dead. Telling a client that her husband won't be able to visit or she will have to wait and see if he will visit are deceptive responses and should be avoided. Acknowledging what the client may be feeling, and that she misses her husband, directs her to talk about a better remembered event and treats the client respectfully with compassion.

NP = An
CN = Ph/8
CL = An
SA = 6

6. 2. Delirium is reversible if treated and often comes on quickly, as opposed to dementia, which has a slow onset. How much water the client drinks will only have an effect if the delirium is related to dehydration or overhydration. Staying with the client to provide safety is important when the client is at risk for injury, but it does not answer the family member's question.
NP = An
CN = Sa/1
CL = An
SA = 6

7. 1. A client with a change in oxygen saturation is hypoxic. The delirium is related to the low oxygen saturation. Administering oxygen at a low flow rate is the safest for an older adult. This would be the first intervention to see if the oxygen saturation and cognition improve. Administering an intravenous infusion of 5% dextrose or orange juice orally are treatments for clients with low blood glucose. Emergency medical treatment is not necessary until further assessment has been provided.
NP = Im
CN = Ph/8
CL = Ap
SA = 6

8. 2. The appropriate nursing intervention for a client with diabetes who wants to wear a coat indoors is to check the blood sugar. The change in mental status is very likely from low blood sugar. If the blood sugar is low, a source of glucose should be given orally, and the nurse should continue assessment before calling the health care provider.
NP = Im
CN = Sa/1
CL = Ap
SA = 6

Practice Test 3

1. An 81-year-old client who speaks limited English and cannot read or calculate has experienced a decline in mental status over the last year. The best measurement tool for the nurse to use to determine baseline cognitive function is the

   1. Mini-Mental State Exam.
   2. The Clock Drawing test.
   3. The Geriatric Depression Scale.
   4. The Minnesota Multiphasic Personality Exam.

2. When a client is diagnosed with Alzheimer's-like dementia, Stage I, the client and family will need to make many decisions and plans for the future. The nurse should act as an advocate and encourage the client and family to make these plans by urging them to

   1. write an advance directive.
   2. sell the client's property.
   3. move the client to a long-term care facility.
   4. put locks on all of the doors at home so the client cannot open them.

3. A 76-year-old widowed client lives alone, is suspicious of strangers, and does not recognize the grandchildren. Occasionally the client goes outside and cannot find the door to reenter the house. The family asks the nurse what could be wrong with the client. Which of the following is the best initial response by the nurse?

   1. "The client spends too much time alone and may benefit from more socialization."

120

2. "It is the beginning of Alzheimer's disease, and different living arrangements should be considered."

3. "A complete medical and psychiatric evaluation should be performed to determine the cause."

4. "It could be the result of a vitamin deficiency."

4. Which of the following interventions is priority for the nurse to implement to prevent incontinence in a client in Stage I Alzheimer's-like dementia?

   1. Toilet the client on a schedule of every two hours when awake

   2. Restrict fluid intake before bedtime

   3. Label all of the bathrooms on the nursing unit with large signs that read "Bathroom"

   4. Use disposable briefs on the client

5. A 76-year-old client who resides in a nursing home is in Stage III of Alzheimer's-like dementia. The family members do not visit the client even though they live in the vicinity. The nurse understands that this lack of contact may be most likely related to

   1. feelings of loss because the older adult does not recognize the family.

   2. the client's aggression toward the family.

   3. the fear of old age and dying.

   4. confusion about nursing home policy.

6. A client in Stage II Alzheimer's-like dementia is resistant to direction from the nurse in the long-term care facility. When asked about the desire to eat, the client's response is always "No." The best plan for eliciting cooperation would be for the nurse to

   1. ask the client twice about the desire to eat, and if the response is "No" do not offer a meal.

   2. provide the client frequent high-calorie snacks.

   3. assist the client to the dining room, stating that there is something there to see.

   4. tell the client it is time to eat and provide a nonstimulating atmosphere with frequent prompts to eat.

7. Tacrine (Cognex) is prescribed for a client in Stage I Alzheimer's-like dementia. The client has become uncooperative, agitated, and more confused since first taking the drug. The nurse should report these behaviors as

   1. an acceleration of the disease process.

   2. adverse reactions to the drug.

    3. the client is not taking the drug.

    4. a larger dose of the drug may be needed.

8. The nurse should assess for which of the following problems as signs of depression in the older adult?

    1. Unexpected diaphoresis

    2. Change of jobs

    3. Bradycardia

    4. Giving away prized possessions

9. Which of the following is the priority nursing diagnosis for an older adult client with dementia and malnutrition who is prone to falling in the hospital?

    1. Confusion, acute

    2. Imbalanced nutrition: less than body requirements

    3. Role performance, ineffective

    4. Risk for injury

10. The daughter of an 83-year-old client with dementia asks the nurse, "Why can't I get my father to eat? He doesn't like his favorite food anymore." What is the best initial response for the nurse to make?

    1. "Do you feel rejected because he doesn't eat your cooking?"

    2. "Why do you think he isn't getting enough to eat?"

    3. "Tell me about your meals and what your father eats."

    4. "Have you considered putting your father in a nursing home?"

11. The wife of an older adult with dementia asks the nurse whether she can spend the night with her husband in the nursing home where he lives. The nurse asks the wife, "Do you have any particular concerns about leaving your husband here tonight?" The wife replies that her husband is very sad and she doesn't want him to be alone. Which of the following is the priority response by the nurse?

    1. "It's against nursing home policy for you to stay at night."

    2. "Your husband doesn't know who you are anymore, so don't stay and tire yourself."

    3. "I will check on your husband more often during the night and spend extra time with him."

    4. "Is there some reason you doubt the quality of care the staff is providing your husband?"

12. Which of the following should the nurse plan for when assessing an older client with dementia for a pain response?

1. Use a visual analog scale for pain assessment
2. Monitor the client for changes in behavior and nonverbal indications of pain
3. Rely on the client's family to tell the nurse if the client is in pain
4. Avoid assessing for pain because the neurological changes prevent the sensation of pain

13. A 77-year-old man with dementia who is a resident in a nursing home dementia unit is trying to open a window and climb out. The client tells the nurse, "I just have to have a soda. I have to get out of here to get one. Don't try to stop me!" In this situation it is essential that the nurse keep the client from harm. When intervening in this situation, the nurse should

    1. restrain the client.
    2. administer haloperidol (Haldol) to the client.
    3. ask the client to sit down and drink a soda with you.
    4. ask the why he wants a soda.

14. Fluoxetine (Prozac) for depression and tacrine (Cognex) for early onset Stage I Alzheimer's-like dementia have been prescribed for an older client. Which of the following should the nurse include in this client's plan of care?

    1. Question the orders for these drugs because a client with dementia may not also be depressed
    2. Check with the prescriber because the drugs interact
    3. Administer the drugs as prescribed
    4. Observe the client carefully for potentiation of the Prozac by the Cognex

15. A client with Stage I Alzheimer's-like dementia asks the nurse, "Because I have Alzheimer's disease, does that mean my children will get it too?" Which of the following is the best response that represents current medical research?

    1. "No, Alzheimer's disease does not run in families."
    2. "You are concerned about your children?"
    3. "Research studies indicate a genetic link to Alzheimer's disease, but that does not mean that your children will get it."
    4. "Don't worry. There are new breakthroughs every day."

16. An older adult client asks the nurse, "Why does my physician say I have Alzheimer's-like dementia? I thought it was Alzheimer's disease." The best response is

1. "They are the same conditions."

2. "Actual Alzheimer's disease can only be diagnosed with an autopsy of the brain."

3. "Why do you want to know the difference?"

4. "I do not know. You will have to ask your physician."

17. Based on an understanding of the medical diagnosis of Stage III Alzheimer's-like dementia, the nurse should plan care for this client based on

    1. the ability of the client to care for self with some memory loss.

    2. an ability to complete an advance directive.

    3. an inability to care for self.

    4. an ability to provide some care with a moderate disability.

18. The registered nurse is planning nursing assignments for a geriatric mental health unit. Which of the following assignments should the nurse delegate to a licensed practical nurse?

    1. Instruct the family of a client with dementia on the course of the illness

    2. Develop a plan of care for an older adult with Alzheimer's disease

    3. Perform a cognitive test on a client with dementia

    4. Administer tacrine (Cognex) to a client with Alzheimer's disease

ANSWERS AND RATIONALES

1. **2.** Even though the Mini-Mental State Exam is considered a valid measure of cognitive function, clients taking it must be able to read and calculate. The Clock Drawing test does not require literacy or a comprehension of English.
   NP = Im
   CN = Ph/8
   CL = An
   SA = 6

2. **1.** In Alzheimer's-like dementia, Stage I, the client is still mostly cognitively intact and capable of making decisions about advance directives, durable power of attorney for health care, and end-of-life care. The nurse should not make decisions for the client or family. Long-term care is not indicated.
   NP = Im
   CN = Ph/8
   CL = Ap
   SA = 6

3. 3. A client who is confused and does not recognize the door of the house is not safe in the current environment and needs a medical and psychiatric evaluation to determine the cause of the altered mental status. The nurse should not diagnose by telling the family the client has Alzheimer's disease or a vitamin deficiency and should encourage the family to provide the safest environment for the client.
NP = An
CN = Sa/1
CL = An
SA = 6

4. 1. A client in Stage I of dementia should be able to indicate the need to eliminate. A toileting schedule will provide needed consistency and prevent incontinence. Labeling all of the bathrooms with large signs may encourage the client to enter inappropriate bathrooms. Disposable briefs should be used as a last resort and in stages II and III of the illness.
NP = Im
CN = Sa/1
CL = An
SA = 8

5. 1. As the client with dementia declines, the family may feel that because the client no longer recognizes them and is unable to interact, contact is not needed. Or, the family may feel a profound sense of loss because the loved one is no longer the same. It is unlikely that in Stage III the client would be aggressive. The fear of old age and dying may be a concern of the family, but is not the most likely cause for the family's avoidance.
NP = An
CN = Ph/8
CL = An
SA= 6

6. 4. In Stage II Alzheimer's-like dementia, the client may not recognize hunger. Asking a yes-or-no question may elicit a "no" response all of the time. In a quiet, nonstimulating environment, the client can attend to eating. The nurse can prompt the client by saying, "This is your spoonful of cereal," or by providing finger foods that do not require skill in manipulating utensils.
NP = Pl
CN = Ph/8
CL = Ap
SA = 6

7. 2. Tacrine (Cognex) is used in the treatment of mild to moderate Alzheimer's-like dementia. Adverse reactions to Cognex include agitation,

dizziness, and confusion. The drug should not be given in a larger dose to see if the behaviors diminish. Alzheimer's-like dementia is a slowly progressing disease.
NP = An
CN = Ph/8
CL = An
SA = 5

8. 4. Diaphoresis may be related to physiological problems or drugs. Changing a job may be the result of the depression and not the cause for the depression. Giving away prized possessions may be an indicator of depression and the client's intention of self-harm.
NP = As
CN = Ph/8
CL = Ap
SA = 6

9. 4. The priority nursing diagnosis for a client who has dementia, is malnourished, and is prone to falling is risk for injury. Although acute confusion, imbalanced nutrition: less than body requirements, and ineffective role performance may all be appropriate nursing diagnoses, they are not the priority. Safety is always the priority.
NP = Ev
CN = Sa/1
CL = Ap
SA = 6

10. 3. The best response to a family member who is concerned that her father does not eat anymore is to further assess the client's food pattern. Asking the family member to tell the nurse about the meals and what the client eats opens communication and leads to more information.
NP = An
CN = Ph/8
CL = An
SA = 6

11. 3. The priority response for a client's wife who wants to spend the night with the client is to tell the wife her husband will be checked on more frequently during the night. It provides emotional support for the client and his wife.
NP = An
CN = Sa/1
CL = An
SA = 6

12. 2. The nurse must be vigilant in observing the client for changes in behavior that would indicate pain, such as rubbing a body part. It would

not be appropriate to use a visual analog scale, because it requires the client to have the ability to think abstractly. It would not be appropriate for the nurse to ask the family about the pain, because the client may not have family available at all times or the family might not know the client's needs. A client with dementia will be able to feel pain, but may not be able to verbalize the degree and location of the pain.
NP = Pl
CN = Ph/8
CL = Ap
SA = 6

13. 3. Chemical and physical restraints are last resorts. Asking clients with dementia why they want a soda will cause a defensive reaction, because the clients cannot rationalize "why." The nurse should redirect the client, and offering a soda draws the client away from the window. Safety is the priority.
NP = Im
CN = Ph/8
CL = Ap
SA = 6

14. 3. Fluoxetine (Prozac) is a selective serotonin reuptake inhibitor antidepressant that may be administered with tacrine (Cognex), which is given in the treatment of mild or moderate Alzheimer's disease. There are no known interactions between Cognex and Prozac. It is possible for a client to have depression and dementia. In Stage I of dementia, a client is aware of the functional losses and may be depressed because of the expected decline from the dementia.
NP = Pl
CN = Ph/8
CL = Ap
SA = 6

15. 3. Research studies indicate there is a genetic link to Alzheimer's disease, but that does not mean the children of a client will get it.
NP = An
CN = Ph/8
CL = An
SA = 6

16. 2. Alzheimer's disease can only be diagnosed with an autopsy of the brain. Providing information to the client is within the scope of practice of the nurse.
NP = An
CN = Ph/8
CL = An
SA = 6

17. 3. Stage III Alzheimer's-like dementia is the end stage of the dementia. Clients are no longer able to remember themselves or family. Clients are not competent to make decisions about care and will require total nursing care.
NP = Pl
CN = Ph/8
CL = Ap
SA = 6

18. 4. A licensed practical nurse may administer a drug to a client with Alzheimer's disease. Providing instructions to a client's family, performing a cognitive test, and developing a plan of care are tasks reserved for the registered nurse.
NP = Pl
CN = Sa/1
CL = An
SA = 8